IS STRESS COMPROMISING YOUR HEALTH
AND DISRUPTING YOUR LIFE?
YOU MIGHT CONSIDER . . .

- **Laughing**—that's right: laughter has actually been shown to release endorphins (the hormones that make us feel good) and decrease the level of stress hormones
- **Rewarding yourself**—scheduling at least one fun or pleasurable activity a day will not only reduce stress, it will make the rest of your day more enjoyable
- **Avoiding foods that aggravate stress**, such as sugars, fats, caffeine and alcohol
- **Taking vitamins, minerals and herbs** that help with stress, such as Vitamin B, calcium, and chamomile
- **Relaxing** with one of the many techniques that promote relaxation, such as deep breathing, meditation, or aromatherapy

FIND OUT MORE SECRETS TO A
STRESS-LESS LIFE IN
**STRESS: 63 WAYS TO RELIEVE TENSION
AND STAY HEALTHY**

Stress:
63 WAYS TO RELIEVE THE TENSION AND STAY HEALTHY

CHARLES B. INLANDER AND CYNTHIA K. MORAN

A People's Medical Society Book

St. Martin's Paperbacks

Published by arrangement with Walker Publishing Company, Inc.

STRESS: 63 WAYS TO RELIEVE TENSION AND STAY HEALTHY

Library of Congress Catalog Card Number: 96-9901

ISBN: 0-312-97399-3

Printed in the United States of America

Walker Publishing Company trade paperback edition published in 1996
St. Martin's Paperbacks edition / June 2000

St. Martin's Paperbacks are published by St. Martin's Press, 175 Fifth Avenue, New York, NY 10010.

10 9 8 7 6 5 4 3 2 1

CONTENTS

INTRODUCTION

I learned firsthand about stress when I was in college. One morning in my junior year, I woke up and my left side was numb. I could use my arm and leg, but I couldn't feel them. My fingers tingled, as did my toes. I went to the university health service, where the doctor couldn't find anything wrong. He sent me to a specialist, who gave me a battery of tests that also came up negative. He gave me some tranquilizers, which didn't solve the problem.

Finally, in my worry, I flew home and visited our family physician. He looked over the test results, ordered a few more, and asked me to return in three days. When I did, he sat me down and said there was nothing organically wrong. He asked what was going on at school. I told him I was taking a full course load, planning all the university concerts, trying to line up a summer job, and working on a variety of university publications. He looked me straight in the eye and said I was doing too much. He told me my symptoms were real, but they were caused by stress. He suggested I cut back on my activities and give myself time to relax. And right there in his office, he taught me several deep-breathing exercises. Amazingly, by the time I walked out of his door, my "left side disease" went away.

Over the years, I have been able to recognize many other symptoms that are stress related. And I have learned strategies and methods to prevent or alleviate those signs of stress. But most people never learn enough about dealing with and conquering the effects of stress. That's why we have written this book.

This book is different from most other books that deal with stress. While they usually teach or preach one technique or method, this book is a compendium of stress prevention strategies and stress busters from experts all over the world. And that's important. No single stress plan works for everyone. That's why the more you know, the better you will be able to handle the stress in your own life.

Medical research has shown that stress is a major cause of disease and illness. It can limit activity, cause severe depression, and even kill. But it is controllable. And we at the People's Medical Society are pleased that we can help you take control of your own life and keep the effects of stress in check.

Charles B. Inlander, President
People's Medical Society

1

UNDERSTANDING STRESS

The American Medical Association defines stress as any interference that disturbs a person's mental and physical well-being. However, we commonly define stress as a response to conditions and events, both routine and out of the ordinary.

The toll stress takes on the nation's health and finances is daunting. National Institute for Mental Health studies and other surveys show that:

- Seventy to 80 percent of all visits to the doctor are for stress-related and stress-induced illnesses.
- People who live in a high state of anxiety are 4.5 times more likely to die of a heart attack or stroke.
- Stress contributes to 50 percent of all illnesses in the United States.
- Stress-related injuries on the job climbed from 5 percent of all occupational disease claims in 1980 to more than 15 percent in 1990.
- The cost of job stress in the United States is estimated at $200 billion annually, including costs

of absenteeism, lost productivity, and insurance claims.

• Seven of 10 respondents to a national poll in 1995 said they felt stress in a typical workday, while 43 percent of those interviewed said they suffer noticeable physical and emotional symptoms of burnout.

No one can completely escape the effects of stress. Undoubtedly, stress is a natural part of being human. It's what keeps us alert and bright and, in the misty past, kept us one step ahead of predators and other dangers to our survival. Even today, stress can function as a source of motivation and a catalyst in the problem-solving process. Also keep in mind that not all stress stems from crises and insurmountable obstacles. It can be prompted by events or conditions that create supercharged feelings of motivation or happiness. But the real issue when it comes to your health, according to experts, is long-term or chronic stress. Whether it's brought on by the good or the bad, chronic stress is not good for you.

This book is about beating chronic stress: how to identify it, why it hurts you, and how to channel it and manage it in your life.

WHAT CAUSES STRESS?

Twentieth-century life is full of stress. We live in a fast-paced world where technology has made it possible for humans to be active 24 hours a day. While our ancestors were forced to go to bed with the end of daylight, electricity has allowed us to stretch our seeing (and working) hours. Jet travel and telecommunications have linked us globally to other societies and added to the frenetic work pace. With America's reverence for productivity at work, says author Staffan Linder in his work *The Harried Leisure Class*, many people are under increasing pressure to work longer and harder to earn more, often leading to the abandonment of leisure activities and family time.*

Causes of stress are known as stressors. Stressors can be physical or emotional, internally or externally generated. A variety of physical and emotional stimuli, including physical violence and internal conflicts, can cause stress. Stress may emanate from major life events—putting an elderly parent in a nursing home, a birth or death, a divorce or marriage—or from more pedestrian fare, such as bouncing a check, getting stuck in a traffic jam, or having a computer crash.

WHAT IS THE STRESS RESPONSE?

The physiological process that occurs when the body first reacts to a stressor has been passed down intact from our earliest ancestors. This "fight-or-flight" mechanism, triggered by the autonomic nervous system, can be life-saving in times of danger. The brain releases the stimulating stress hormones cortisol and epinephrine (also known as adrenaline) into the system. The heart beats faster, blood pressure rises, muscles tense, the senses sharpen, and metabolism changes. Blood pumps to the organs most needed to respond to an attack, which leaves the extremities, such as the hands, cold and clammy. The psychological effects are characterized by

---

*New York: Columbia University Press, 1970.

feelings of apprehension, tension, and nervousness.

This reaction happens instantaneously, clearly a help in situations involving an immediate physical danger. But all too often, the "danger" is loss of a job, prolonged illness, death of a loved one. Unfortunately, many modern stressors do not go away quickly, so the body stays primed to react. Continued exposure to stress can lead to mental and physical symptoms, such as anxiety and depression, heart palpitations, and muscle aches and pains. Illness often follows.

Yet it's only recently that we have discovered why.

HOW DID WE FIRST LEARN ABOUT THE BAD EFFECTS OF STRESS?

Stress, the stress response, and the negative effects of chronic stress were first definitively linked in the 1930s when McGill University endocrinologist Hans Selye studied the behavior of rats. Specifically, he observed what happened to rats' hormones when they were subjected to a variety of stressors, including starvation, extremes in temperature, and slamming doors. Along with Walter Cannon, another prominent physiological researcher of the 1930s, Selye applied the engineering term *stress* to define the myriad of traumatizing behaviors to which the rats had been subjected. To explain how they reacted to stress, he coined the term *general adaptation syndrome*, a response, he said, that consists of three stages: alarm, adaptation (or resistance), and exhaustion.*

The first stage occurs, according to Selye, when the

The Stress of Life. New York: McGraw-Hill, 1984.

body becomes aware of the stressor, alerts its systems, then prepares to meet the threat (the fight-or-flight response). The second stage occurs when the body either adapts to the threat or successfully resists the threat with its stress-response mechanism and then returns to its natural, or homeostatic, state. The third stage occurs only after prolonged exposure to stressors and is marked by the stressed body contracting various diseases. Selye attributed this phenomenon to a depletion of the body's stress-response hormones.

Remarkably, much of Selye's original stress research has stood the test of decades. Today, however, we know that the body's stress hormones, cortisol and epinephrine, are not normally depleted. Unfortunately, it is their continued presence that causes damage after prolonged periods of stress. Even though rises in the levels of stress hormones vary from person to person and also according to the degree of stress, there is growing evidence that these hormonal changes may lead to disease.

HOW ARE BODILY SYSTEMS AFFECTED BY CHRONIC STRESS?

While the body is on an all-out alert in response to a stressor, breathing is quick and shallow. This depletes the flow of oxygen, which cells need for maintenance and health. The chronic state of readiness also shuts down functions such as metabolism, causing indigestion, heartburn, and decreased sex drive. Stress also takes its toll on the cardiovascular and immune systems. Stress often attacks the body's most vulnerable areas, spots made weak by a past illness or injury or by genetic disposition.

The cardiovascular system is now known to suffer some of the most debilitating effects of chronic stress. Studies in animals have shown that cortisol raises the level of cholesterol and other lipids in the blood and accelerates the development of arteriosclerosis (hardening of the arteries) and other signs of damage to blood vessels. Cardiologist and stress researcher Robert S. Eliot, M.D., uncovered yet another kind of heart damage initiated by stress hormones. He discovered that the presence of excessive cortisol causes lesions in the heart muscles. In his book *From Stress to Strength*, Eliot explains that a mass of lesions, created over time by unchecked stress, ultimately causes the heart's main pumping chambers to overcontract: The heart starts pumping so erratically that without first aid (usually consisting of an electric shock with a defibrillator), death results.* Other negative cardiovascular effects include irregular heart rhythms and chest pain.

Further, research is increasingly showing us the negative effects of stress on the immune system. The body's defense against infection and disease consists of lymphatic vessels, organs (the thymus gland, spleen, tonsils, adenoids, and lymph nodes), white blood cells, specialized cells that live in the tissues, and specialized serums. The hormones triggered by stress are thought to inhibit the activity of white blood cells, the cells that fight off disease, and have also been connected to cancer by some studies. They also shrink the thymus gland, which is responsible for the development and maintenance of the body's immune system. This results in the release of fewer immunizing hormones by the thymus gland during

---

*New York: Bantam, 1994.

periods of undue or prolonged stress. Scientists also believe that the immune system, which works best during relaxation and sleep, suffers during chronic stress, since stress promotes the functions of the body's conscious, voluntary systems.

The effects of stress on the immune system are well documented. In a study on stress and the common cold, researchers at Carnegie Mellon University sprayed cold viruses into the noses of 400 volunteers. They found that those people with high stress in their lives were twice as likely to develop colds. In another study, Ohio State University researchers measured the immune functions of 19 volunteers, each of whom had been caring for a seriously ill spouse, against those of 69 people who had no such obligation. Findings more than a year later showed that the caregivers had significantly weaker primary immune functions than the other group, and their colds lasted twice as long.

An intriguing twist on the stress/immune system connection has emerged as a result of research conducted at the University of Rochester. Previously, researchers believed that the fight-or-flight response caused the destruction of immune cells and weakened the immune response. The newer study demonstrated that a stressful experience deploys immune cells to different parts of the body where they may be needed to attack any invading organisms. Once the stressful situation has passed, the cells migrate back to their normal locations in the body. This may explain why during a major event or crisis people can push themselves and not get sick, only to become ill after the stressful event has passed.

It is important to note here that this finding pertains specifically to short-lived stress. Researchers acknowledge that chronic or long-term stress definitely suppresses the immune response.

CAN STRESS AFFECT THE MIND?

Findings indicate that chronic stress can accelerate memory loss. Recent studies have focused on the effect of stress on the hippocampus, the brain's memory center. One study consisted of administering to animals repeated doses of cortisol, the hormone released in the body during stress. The animals' hippocampi were then measured and found to have lost cells, implying that stress has a negative effect on the hippocampus and therefore on memory.

A six-year Swedish study that measured memory and other mental skills in 130 older men also showed that stress affects memory. In that study, the decline in memory and other mental skills was six times greater in those whose partner or child had died during the study. Other research is beginning to show that stress hormones also overstimulate those areas of the brain most closely linked to depression, which may make people with chronic stress more susceptible to that condition.

HOW CAN WE TELL WHEN STRESS IS BECOMING UNHEALTHY?

What determines whether stress is unhealthy for us is a combination of how much stress we have in our lives at any given moment and how we react to it. A little stress—good or bad—can be beneficial because it keeps us alert, challenges us, and assures us that all of our systems are responding. When stress moves into the harmful category, it can manifest itself as a combination of behavioral, emotional, intellectual, and physical symptoms, which may indicate stress isn't being coped with. Pioneer researcher Selye divided stress symptoms into three categories:

BEHAVIORAL/EMOTIONAL

anger and hostility
apprehension
blaming others
complaining
critical of self to others
crying
defensive behavior
denial
depression
diminished initiative
excessive alcohol use
excessive smoking
gulping meals

habitual teeth grinding
  (bruxism)
indecisiveness
irritability
lack of satisfaction from
  happy experiences
mistrust
mood swings
nail biting
panic
restlessness
suicidal tendencies
withdrawal

INTELLECTUAL

diminished fantasy life
forgetfulness
lack of attention to
  details
lack of awareness of
  external stimuli

lack of concentration
past rather than future
  orientation
preoccupation
reduced creativity

(Continued on next page)

(continued)

PHYSICAL

anorexia	indigestion,
chronic fatigue	stomachaches
constipation	insomnia
cool, clammy skin	itchy scalp
diarrhea	loss of appetite
dilated pupils	nausea and/or vomiting
disturbed motor skills	overeating
dry mouth	rash
frequent urination	sneezing
headaches	spasm of the hands or
heart palpitations	feet
hyperactivity	stooped posture
hyperventilation	sweaty palms
impaired sexual	tight muscles
function	trembling, tics, or
	twitches

IS THERE SUCH A THING AS A STRESS-RESISTANT PERSON?

No one is immune to all stress, but some tolerate it better than others. A landmark study in 1989 initiated by Raymond B. Flannery, M.D., sought to identify the principal qualities needed for stress resistance.* Project SMART, as it was called, studied 1,200 persons who seemed to resist stress well and concluded that the person who effectively resists stress embodies four qualities: (1) looks at problems positively, as challenges to be met; (2) has personal goals that are well defined; (3) engages in a

---

Harvard Medical Letter (February 1989).

sensible lifestyle that includes regular aerobic exercise and a method of relaxation; and (4) is socially involved with others. (To help you evaluate stress in your life, a series of self-tests has been included in the appendix of this book.)

While studies show that some illnesses cannot be helped without some medical intervention as well as a stress management program, there is little doubt that employing regular stress reduction techniques will boost your immunity, improve your outlook, and, overall, make your life a lot more pleasurable. Now let's get started.

2

TIPS FOR PREVENTING AND RELIEVING STRESS

While the bad news is that many illnesses and diseases in America are linked to stress, the good news is that people seem to be getting the message about the importance of trying to prevent and relieve stress. Stress reduction is an effort that requires self-awareness, optimism, assertiveness, and a personal strategy for handling stressful events. It also involves careful attention to your body and your health. Tips in this chapter help you learn how to deal with stress and, more important, how to keep it from finding you in the first place.

LIFESTYLE

The way you live, your attitudes and emotions, and the company you keep all play roles in how much stress you have and how you handle it. Try these tactics to help keep yourself in a stress-free frame of mind.

✓ *Laugh.*

Laughter may be one of the healthiest antidotes to stress, studies show. When we laugh or even, according to some research, when we just smile, blood flow to the brain is increased, endorphins (painkilling hormones that give us a sense of well-being) are released, and levels of stress hormones drop. Research undertaken at Loma Linda University Schools of Medicine and Public Health shows that comedy lowers the body's levels of cortisol and epinephrine, thereby lowering blood pressure and diminishing other cardiovascular problems. The decrease in stress hormones allows an increase in white blood cell production, which increases immunity.

The late author Norman Cousins did breakthrough personal research when he elected to fight his ankylosing spondylitis, a crippling and irreversible form of arthritis, by renting funny movies and laughing as much as possible. His disease went into remission, and he outlived medical expectations.

To achieve stress-free living through laughter, most of us have some serious work to do. A study reported in the July/August 1995 issue of *Men's Health* showed that toddlers laugh an average of 400 times a day while adults manage only 15 chortles.

✓ *Be a social animal.*

When we are under stress, our instincts often tell us to withdraw from the action and isolate ourselves. Nothing could be worse, according to experts, since isolation allows us to concentrate more on our problem(s) and on negative thinking, activities that intensify rather than help resolve stress. Years of research support theories that tie isolation to failure to cope adequately with stress, heightened vulnerability to illness, and even premature death.

Try calling friends to join you for a meal or make a point of being around young children, who have a way of making us forget ourselves and our worries. Or do some rewarding volunteer work. A 10-year University of Michigan study showed that the death rate was twice as high in men who did no volunteer work as in those who volunteered at least once a week.

✓ *Know your stress personality.*
Do you know how you react to stress? Do you yell and kick the furniture when there's too much on your plate? Or do you retreat into stony silence? Keep a stress diary for two weeks. Make note of any stressor—the item or event that causes you stress; the time, place, and day it occurs; how you feel (angry, defeated, tired, over-whelmed); and what you do as a result. By knowing your own personality and triggers, you can learn to respond to stress before you reach crisis mode.

Robert K. Cooper, Ph.D., author of *The Performance Edge*, recommends invoking what he calls the instant calming sequence at the first sign of a stress trigger:*

- Do uninterrupted breathing.
- Put on a positive face. Studies show that optimists are better able to cope with stress than pessimists are.
- Stand in a balanced posture.
- Release muscle tension.

*Boston: Houghton Mifflin, 1991.

• Exert mental control. Focus your thoughts on the situation and your options for solving it.

Tips on posture, breathing, and relaxation methods are discussed later in this chapter.

✓ *Get rid of anger.*

Anger itself is not toxic, but how we express it—or repress it—can be. A University of Michigan School of Public Health study concluded that poorly managed anger is linked to a 2.5 times greater risk of death. The most notable findings in recent stress research indicate that anger, specifically hostility, is the single most damaging stress-related personality trait that precedes a heart attack. One long-term study, discussed in the April 25, 1994, *New York Times*, examined men who took a hostility test while they were law students. Many years later the follow-up study revealed that almost 20 percent of those in the top quarter of the hostility scale had died by the age of 50, compared with only 4 percent of those in the lowest quarter of the scale.

What's the best way to deal with anger? Conventional wisdom holds that it is healthy to vent rage in order to get it out in the open. On the other hand, Cooper recommends "reflective coping"—acknowledging anger without resorting to open physical or verbal hostility. Discuss the conflict with the other person or sort things out on your own; either helps you to avoid hostility and regain emotional control. Those who practice reflective coping, says Cooper, solve problems faster and more effectively, get the anger out of their systems, and have superior health to those who harbor a grudge or explode. For the same reasons, many stress experts recommend an exercise in "forgiveness therapy": After a hostile situation has been settled (or even if it hasn't been), letting bygones be bygones can bring closure and reduce anger to indifference, reducing stress levels.

✓ *Make your job work for you.*
A recent survey by Northwestern National Life showed that while workers blame overwork for job dissatisfaction, the real cause of their job-related stress is a lack of personal control. A Bureau of National Affairs study found that as many as one in four bosses manages the office the way his or her parents ran the home, using tactics that demean, insult, or otherwise abuse employees. Not surprisingly, that study showed employees subjected to that kind of control-eroding treatment have more health problems. In another study that examined all jobs in the Volvo plant in Göteborg, Sweden, those who saw themselves as influential were more highly motivated and less subject to stress-related medical complaints than those who saw themselves as cogs in the wheel.

In his pioneering work on stress and job rank, industrial engineer Robert Karasek, now at the University of California, Berkeley, concluded that the most stressful position is not at the top. He found that the more heart-attack-prone, higher-stress posts belong to secretaries and lower-ranking workers in high-demand areas with low control rather than to CEOs, who have a high degree of control in their jobs.

While you probably can't rewrite your company's culture, you can change the way you react to issues of control on the job. Here are some tips:

- Try to be an active participant. Passivity leads to stress and lack of personal control. Ask and answer questions, attend company meetings and events, and be sure your voice is heard in the workplace.

- Be supportive of coworkers. Social support works as a palliative. Good relationships with peers, with a respectful boss, or with members of a team on which you participate help to establish a sense of control of some part of your job.

- When your loss of control is precipitated by an upsetting event, try counting to 10 before you react. This helps avoid conflict, and the pause can help you regain a sense of control.

- If you know you are in the wrong job, accept the fact and consider improving your skills during leisure time so that you can change jobs (or even career paths).

THE PLAGUE OF JOB STRESS

The link between your occupation, stress, and depression is very strong. A 1990 Johns Hopkins University study of 12,000 workers showed a high correlation between stress and how much autonomy—control—a worker feels he or she has.

The highest-stress job categories include the following: lawyers, secretaries, data entry and computer operators, special education teachers and school counselors, typists, health aides, waiters and waitresses, food preparation workers, and sales personnel. All do demanding work for which others set the rules. In today's downsized corporate America, where one worker is often doing the jobs that 3.1 persons did a decade ago, task demand is even more intense than it was during the 1990 Hopkins study. In spite of this reality, business writer Morty Lefkoe, quoted in *The Wellness Encyclopedia*, reports that some businesses create lower stress by organizing work around self-determined commitments, showing equality in titles, encouraging trust and open communication, and paying high attention to the safety and security of their employees.* University of California, Berkeley, researchers Robert Karasek and Tores Theorell, also in *The Wellness Encyclopedia*, conclude that seven key ingredients make up job satisfaction:

- Skill discretion. This allows maximum use of skills and a chance to improve or increase skills.
- Autonomy. Control over what it is that you do may include participation in long-term planning and flexible hours.
- Psychological demands. Old routines are mixed with new. There are predictable challenges, and workers have some say in demands made on them.
- Social relations. Workers can collaborate.
- Social rights. Democratic procedures rule, and grievance procedures are in place.
- Meaningfulness. Employees understand what they are producing and for whom and get feedback from customers.
- Integration of family and community life with work. Their jobs allow employees time and energy for family responsibilities and activities outside of work.

---

*University of California, Berkeley. Boston: Houghton Mifflin, 1991.

✔ *Be decisive.*
Indecision prevents you from taking action, causing a loss of a sense of control and thus intensifying stress. If you're indecisive, how can you adapt your behavior? First, write down the problem and a list of your options, including the option of doing nothing, suggests stress researcher Leon Chaitow, D.O., in his book *Stress.** Then, he says, rather than doing linear thinking (starting at a given point and moving toward a desired objective), try lateral thinking, in which you consider unusual alternatives and their pros and cons. Further, be ready to compromise. It helps to remember there's hardly a decision made that can't be modified at a later point.

✔ *Be assertive.*
Stand up for your decisions. Many people incorrectly equate assertiveness with hostility and aggressiveness, but instead it simply means expressing your feelings, letting others know your beliefs and opinions about something, and acting on your own behalf to satisfy your beliefs and needs. Psychologist James W. Mills, Ph.D., in *Coping With Stress*, suggests these ways to become more assertive: Speak up, start conversations, seek out and initiate a friendship, disagree with others when you believe differently, give as well as accept compliments, ask for information, tell someone else

*London: Thorsons, 1995.

about yourself, and make your wishes and needs
known to others.*

✓ Break the stress-sleeplessness cycle.

Lack of adequate sleep—on average, an adult needs between seven and eight hours a night—can make you
moody, angry, and more vulnerable to illness and the
daily stressors that stalk you. During sleep, replenish-
ment and repair of cells take place, the immune system
is fortified, toxins are filtered out of the body, and muscles relax. The National Commission on Sleep Disorders
found that 36 percent of us do not get enough sleep.
Along with stress, fatigue ranks among the top five reasons people see a doctor.†

If you wake up an hour or two after bedtime with
your mind churning over office or family matters, here
are some tips to help relieve your problem:

- Develop a daily sleep routine, or ritual, that signals
  your mind it's time to sleep.
- Don't drink alcohol or caffeine and don't smoke.
  These all have negative effects on sleep.
- Do something calming before bed. Don't watch a
  violence-filled movie or read an intricately plotted
  book, such as a murder mystery.
- Reserve your bedroom for sleeping and sex only.
- During the day, but especially before bed, practice
  a relaxation strategy. (See the "Self-Care" section
  of this chapter for more information on relaxation
  strategies.)

---

*New York: John Wiley and Sons, 1994.
†*Newsweek* (March 6, 1995).

✔ *Adapt your environment.*

Color, lighting, and noise are all elements that engage and influence our senses. They can work against you, adding stress—or for you, as environmental stress reducers.

• **Color.** Psychologist Max Luscher, Ph.D., did pioneering work on the psychology of color, theorizing that our color response, just like the stress response, harks back to earliest times. To reduce stress in your surroundings, paint a room a pale blue—considered by color theorists to be a calming color—or pure white (with colorful accessories) rather than a bright, aggressive color that's more apt to keep you stressed.

• **Light.** The kind of indoor lighting in which you live and work can play a major role in stress. If there are harsh fluorescent lights that bother you, try going from a cool blue tint to a warm-hued bulb. Some migraine sufferers avoid fluorescent lighting altogether, since its subliminal flickering is thought to trigger migraines. If for whatever reason you can't change the fluorescent lights, add an incandescent lamp to the area to help offset the glare overhead.

The advent of the VDT, the computer monitor, has focused our attention on light and eye problems. VDTs should never be backlit (set against a window, for example) because the glare is potentially damaging to eyesight. Nor should a monitor be positioned so that it reflects any indoor light. Avoid squinting, which tightens the head and neck muscles and changes the blood flow to your head, both stress inducers. Finally, no matter what lighting you work in, take "eye breaks" on a routine basis. If you're doing computer work, try to take a five-minute break—change your focus and look far away, then move your head around—at least once an hour, if not more often.

• **Noise.** A noisy environment is a stressful environment. Besides damaging hearing, it can speed the heart rate, affect mood, prevent concentration or clear thinking, and contribute to nervous disorders.

The Occupational Safety and Health Administration considers 70 decibels of noise the average maximum level for long-term safe exposure. Safety (which takes into account healthy stress levels), say *Office Biology* authors Edith Weiner and Arnold Brown, decreases substantially with every 5-decibel increase.* For your comparison: An overhead plane rates 110 to 120 decibels; a phone bell, 800; traffic, 70 to 90; and a noisy restaurant, 70.

The fact is, it doesn't even have to be loud noise to add to your stress level. Background noise counts, too. One of the most damaging and ubiquitous workplace noises, for instance, may be the low-frequency humming of an air-filtering machine or air conditioner, a computer or copying machine, or even an overhead fluorescent light.

Research shows that we are stressed and physiologically bothered by noises even when we think we don't hear them anymore. One study conducted near an airport monitored sleeping volunteers who claimed they had grown so accustomed to the noise of landing aircraft that they didn't even hear it anymore. The findings proved differently: These people had far more fragmented

---

*New York: MasterMedia, 1994.

sleep—resulting in fatigue, weakened immune systems, and more stress—than those who did not live near such intrusive noise.

✔ *Encourage yourself.*

If you're usually (or always) inclined to blame yourself for your problems—even when they are not your fault—you may be guilty of negative self-talk, which is a stress maker. Instead, try talking positively to yourself—in front of a mirror for practice, if necessary. Tell yourself "Good job" or "You handled that tough situation well." Eventually, positive talk becomes an automatic response. Studies show that those who accept mishaps as largely routine and normal occurrences in life and who talk to themselves in positive terms about these events have higher self-esteem and much lower stress levels.

✔ *Choose winners.*

Relationships take time and a great deal of emotional energy, so invest wisely when developing and maintaining a close relationship, whether in friendship, love, or business. Negative, hypercritical, or isolated people add stress to any relationship. Conversely, people who are optimistic, have high self-esteem, and seek the company of others tend to have less stress and contribute to lower stress levels in those around them.

✔ *Reward yourself.*

Rewards—acknowledgments of task benchmarks—are a critical component of stress management. They have the positive physiological consequence of releasing endorphins, the hormones that reduce pain and help make us feel good—thereby relieving stress. Important research has now confirmed further benefits of regular rewards: A study at the State University of New York at Stony Brook, reported by psychologist Arthur Stone, Ph.D., showed that those who reward themselves by engaging in something pleasurable realize a boost in the disease-fighting quality of their immune systems for several days.

What sorts of rewards are we suggesting? Any activities or situations that you enjoy or that make you smile, and they need not cost much money: going to the movies, browsing in a favorite bookstore, spending time with a good friend, visiting your favorite pond or city park, reading a favorite magazine, placing a 10-minute phone call to a friend . . . the list is endless.

If you can't take time out for a real reward at work, at least give yourself a small pat on the back with a 10-minute mind break (walk around the office, do relaxation exercises, eat a healthy snack). Follow up with something special at the end of the workday. Incidentally, a good stress management technique is scheduling at least one enjoyable activity per day, whether or not you're in the reward business.

✔ *Establish rituals.*
A ritual is an established procedure, system, pattern, or practice. People who have a lot of stress in their lives often tend to live surrounded by mental and physical chaos. Establishing rituals can help prevent and reduce stress by saving time. Important activities are done in a regular and consistent manner, and because rituals become second nature, there is little forethought needed to decide how and when to undertake an activity. Also, a

ritual can be a comfort factor in times of stress, when predictability and certainty reassure us that no matter how bad conditions get, some things remain constant.

✓ *Nurture your spirituality.*
Religious or spiritual beliefs give us a context larger than ourselves, which can provide us with perspective when we are deeply stressed. Those with strong faith often say they derive the strength to face tragedy or huge problems from their beliefs. Research has tended to find that faith in a higher power can help us relieve stress. In his book *Why Zebras Don't Get Ulcers*, author Robert M. Sapolsky, Ph.D., recounts a study of parents of young children terminally ill with cancer.* The parents who felt that God was choosing them—and their child—to carry a special burden were likely to respond better to stress than those who rejected spirituality.

Spirituality needn't take place in a formal place of worship. It may mean no more than communing with nature on a daily walk in the woods or taking quiet, reflective time out of your day to contemplate something more than life's mundane stresses. However, organized religion provides the structures of ritual and ceremony, both of which lend firm support and can be calming in a time of stress. Notes Mills in *Coping With Stress*, rituals and ceremonies, established by societies and religions for the most crucial moments in life (graduations, weddings, and funerals, for example), bring us into contact with others, provide us with guides on how to react, and help us share the experience and wisdom of others.

---

*New York: W. H. Freeman, 1995.

✓ Pen pent-up emotions.

Writing down your feelings in a diary may help relieve emotional stress caused by losing a job, suffering marital problems, being angry at a friend or family member, or enduring other traumatic experiences. This is especially helpful for those who have trouble talking about a problem, worry, or deeply emotional issue. It's also for those people who have no readily available listeners.

Some experts feel the simple act of disclosure is what helps relieve stress. In one study, conducted by psychologist James W. Pennebaker, Ph.D., of Southern Methodist University, participants wrote for 20 minutes a day over four consecutive days about issues or emotions that were causing them stress. Those who stuck to the exercise showed improved mental health and were better able to cope with stress.

✓ Frown on perfection.

Do you delay starting projects because you know they won't be done perfectly? Are you highly anxious about doing every project just right? Do you work, then polish, then polish again until you finally miss your deadline?

If you do, then you have a perfectionist streak, a habit that fuels a whole variety of stress-producing qualities, including procrastination, defensiveness, fear, guilt, and failure to delegate. One study reviewed reports from 9,000 managers and professionals and concluded that perfectionism results in reduced job performance. The research also cited health problems that result from this form of self-induced stress. In addition, those who set their standards unachievably high tend to lose self-esteem when they fail to meet their goals, which only adds to stress.

Defeating perfectionism demands taking charge of what's on your agenda, whether it's at work or at home. Decide how much time you have, then analyze what degree of quality must be embodied in the finished project. Sometimes it's not necessary to do a project of top quality when one of lesser quality will suffice. (Some call this suboptimization.) Once you've set these parameters, get started and follow through.

✔ *Be a kid.*

The next time you're feeling anxious or stressed, take a break and go back to your childhood. Do something goofy: Find crayons and draw a picture, rent a favorite childhood movie, revisit the five-and-ten to buy a bubble-blowing kit (then use it), borrow some fun children's books or find a few old favorites. A day of revisiting times when life was simpler is a good, inexpensive stress buster. Having fun, just like laughing, prompts a release of endorphins, the feel-good hormones.

Workplaces have picked up on the goofy theme, too. The June 16, 1994, *Wall Street Journal* reported on a California ad agency that places punching bags, decorated with the faces of its executives, in its club room. The same agency encourages staff members to paint their offices in wild colors. Another held an indoor golf tournament on two nine-hole courses the employees had constructed.

✔ *Slow down.*

Try moving, talking, and behaving in a relaxed, slower manner and see if it doesn't let some of your stress ebb away. Stephan Rechtschaffen, M.D., director of the Omega Institute for Holistic Studies, suggests these slow-down tips:*

- Drive 10 miles per hour slower. Pay special attention if you drive fast even when you're not rushing.
- Pause at the table before you eat. Saying grace or just sitting quietly, says Rechtschaffen, makes us appreciate food instead of simply wolfing it down. When you eat, consciously chew your food more slowly than usual.
- Wait five minutes in your driveway before entering your house. Listen to your radio, or don't. But relax, chill out, and ease into the transition to home.
- Take an after-work shower. It's relaxing, and it signals a change from your work environment.
- Let the phone ring a few times before answering. Racing across the room to get it on the first ring triggers stress all over again.

✓ *Be a pet person.*

Whether it's a dog, cat, bird, fish, hamster, or guinea pig, a pet can play a vital role in stress relief. A Johns Hopkins Medical Center study found that 50 out of 53 people with pets were alive a year after their first heart attacks, while only 17 of 39 of those without pets lived the year. A 12-month University of California, Los Angeles, study of Medicare enrollees showed that the third who owned pets visited their doctors less than the pet-free group did.

Why the great track record? Doctors suggest that peo-

Psychology Today (November/December 1993).

ple develop emotional bonds with their pets, and bonding helps keep loneliness and stress at bay. And pets give us something else to think about when we are stressed.

✔ *Prepare for changes and minimize uncertainty.*

Research has shown that if a person knows how bad a predicted occurrence will be, he or she will experience less of a stress response than someone who knows *only* to expect something bad to happen. Further, just lack of predictability is apparently enough to cause stress. In *Why Zebras Don't Get Ulcers*, Sapolsky recounts the study of a caged rat that received food delivered down a chute at regular intervals. Changing the predictable pattern of food delivery—giving the same amount of food but in a random fashion—elevated the rat's stress level, despite the fact that the rat faced no other stress. So learn as much as you can about the stressful situation you are facing or about to face. Then anticipate how you'll react to the potentially stressful event when it occurs. Act out your response with a friend or talk to yourself while looking in a mirror. Then once the stressful situation arises, you'll be able to switch to stress-lowering automatic pilot. Studies show that when a familiar stressor is repeated, it triggers a milder stress response.

Another way to minimize uncertainty is to avoid voluntary change during times of stress. Make only the changes you must and defer what's elective—such as moving into a new house—until you bring your stress level back under control. Change can be healthy, but it may hold surprises. You need to remember that stress is cumulative and that even good stress adds to your stress total.

✓ Take vacations.

The true meaning of vacation derives from the word *vacant*: a time that is empty or unscheduled. It's an ideal time to gain perspective on your day-to-day life and to put aside the stress load for a few days. Stress experts say it's important to get a total change of scenery, a new environment, on vacation. Workers who use their vacations to work at home are not recharging nearly as well as they would if they were away from home for the same period.

Statistics show an alarmingly few American workers are taking bona fide vacations, when they take them at all. In their poll of 11,000 people, *Prevention* editors found that one of four who answered took no vacation at all. Those in the survey's low-stress group averaged 2.2 weeks of vacation per year, while those in the high-stress group took 1.4 weeks a year. "A lot of people are working 24 hours a day, seven days a week, even when they're technically not at work," said Boston University Medical Center's Mark Moskowitz, M.D.* Moskowitz calls it a formula for exhaustion.

✓ Get a hobby.

A hobby has been defined as hard work you wouldn't do for a living. If you pursue a hobby you genuinely like, you're apt to get so absorbed in it that you don't notice time passing. You'll forget stress and reach a level

---

Newsweek (March 6, 1995).

of total relaxation. If you are hobby-less, think about a leisure activity that challenges the mind. Further, try to pick something that doesn't add frustration to your stress. For instance, if you are nonathletic, golf or tennis is probably not for you.

Hobbies also help add balance and diversity to our lives. Look at your professional life and choose something very different. For example, if your work deals largely in intangibles, pick a tangible hobby that allows you to see the results, such as ceramics, painting, or woodworking. If you work under constant deadline pressure, choose an open-ended activity with no time line: roller skating, hiking, or making models. If you work alone, try joining a hobby club or taking up a team sport.

TIME MANAGEMENT

Most people think of stress in terms of "So much to do, so little time." If you always seem to be one step behind, try these strategies for getting organized and getting things done.

✓ *Define your limits, then say no.*
Limits, says psychotherapist Lynn Weiss, Ph.D., define how you take charge of your time and space and get in touch with your feelings.* They express the extent of your responsibility and power and show others what you are willing to do or accept. Without limits, it's difficult to say no, which only invites stress when you're involved in more than you can handle.

---

*The Attention Deficit Disorder in Adults Workbook. Dallas: Taylor, 1994.

If after defining your limits you still have trouble saying no, try this four-step strategy:†

- **Stop.** Resist the temptation to answer right away; instead, say "I'll have to let you know tomorrow."
- **Weigh the request against your values and your goals.** How important is it in the context of your life? Is it more important than goal-related tasks you're already doing?
- **Decide.**
- **Respond.** If you're apt to get tongue-tied, write answers down first. If you say no, be willing to explain how you came to your decision, using your goal and value framework—"I have other priorities taking all of my time right now, and I wouldn't be able to give good attention to your request." This also shows the other person you're not being arbitrary.

✓ *Set short-term goals and prioritize them.*

How many times have you heard someone groan "I just don't know where to begin"? A large project, whether it's painting the house or preparing your company's annual report, can be overwhelming, making it tough to get started or make much headway. If this happens, compartmentalize the chores, maybe even assigning time frames for completion. Spreading out the tasks gives you some perspective on the whole and allows you to feel a sense of accomplishment at each step.

Once your goals are clear, set priorities. This means

---

†Xerox Learning Systems. *Help Yourself Time Management*. Stamford, Conn.: Xerox, 1984.

choosing specifically how you spend your time in order to best achieve your objectives. Time management expert Edwin C. Bliss, writing in *Getting Things Done*, defines these categories for reviewing activities:*

- important and urgent (high impact on your objectives and must be done right away)
- important but not urgent (high impact on objectives but may be deferred)
- urgent but not important (little or no impact on objectives but great pressure to do it now)
- busy work (neither urgent nor important but allows you to feel you've accomplished something—usually done when you are avoiding other work)
- wasted time (activities that accomplish nothing)

Another way to evaluate the priority of a chore, Bliss says, is to ask yourself these questions: "Can I save time without sacrificing results if I do this activity less often? If I change the quality of the activity's outcome or the method I use to achieve it? If I don't do it at all?"

Setting priorities is easier if you keep your values in mind. In fact, many stress experts suggest that you begin your fight against stress by defining your values. Start by writing a simple list of qualities you consider important: sense of adventure, wealth, security, meaningful work, serving or helping others, and friendship, for example. Next, think about each in the context of your life. In his book *From Stress to Strength*, cardiologist and stress researcher Robert S. Eliot, M.D., suggests listing up to 10 adjectives that describe how you want to be

---

*New York: Scribners, 1983.

perceived.* Then list 10 a friend would use to describe you and 10 an enemy would use. By comparing the three lists, you can learn whether your current values need fine-tuning or if there are any adjectives on the list you wish were not. Such an evaluation helps you to hold your course when stress hits and make difficult choices when too many things are competing for your attention.

✓ *Delegate.*

Giving responsibilities to others is recognition that you cannot do everything yourself. Those who don't learn to delegate become overloaded with unfinished tasks, making them stressed, less productive, and isolated by their excessive expectations. In his book *Performance Edge*, Cooper suggests that instead of asking yourself "Who can best tackle this or assume responsibility?"—to which you'll probably answer "I can"—you should ask "Who should handle this?" To this question you'll probably answer "Not me."

Once you commit to handing off the task, be absolutely sure both sides understand what needs to be accomplished and any associated deadlines. Establish checkpoints along the way to help reduce your stress, especially if you're a new delegator.

✓ *Be in control of your finances.*

A survey of 11,000 adults in *Prevention* showed the number-one source of stress is worry over personal finances. Research also shows that people trying to maintain lifestyles they can't afford are more likely to have health problems. Here are tips from Michael Ep-

*New York: Bantam, 1994.

stein, M.D., and Sue Hosking's book *Falling Apart* that
may help reduce your stress in this department:*

- Write out your financial goals and your approach
  to getting there.
- Keep all bills and receipts in one place. Set time
  aside each week to pay important bills. If you're
  behind on your bills, try 10 minutes a day until
  you catch up.
- Call on family or friends. Ask for help in organizing your bills or for tips on paying them. Talk
  with them before making any major purchase.
- Make shopping lists. Shop for food only when you
  aren't hungry and for clothing only when you need
  it, and stay within your budget. Do not shop when
  you are depressed.
- Do regular preventive maintenance on your house
  and car.
- Go to a financial counselor for help.
- If you are missing payments on your debt but
  working with a counselor, keep your bank or other
  creditors informed about your situation.

✔ *Sharpen your time management skills.*
In the words of one stress expert, time management is
not about how to cram more into your day. Instead, it's
about using what time you have most beneficially to
reach your personal goals.*
- **Be analytical.** Ask yourself these questions: "Am I
  trying to be accessible to everyone at all times?"

---

*Sebastopol, Calif.: CRCS, 1992.
*Eliot, *From Stress to Strength.*

("People pleasers" seldom move toward their own goals because their time is being controlled by everyone else's goals.) "Does busy work—work that's not important or urgent—give me a feeling of accomplishment?" (If you answer yes, analyze why you are avoiding certain stressful tasks and what you can do to make them more palatable.)

- **Give yourself a pop quiz.** When you're feeling stressed, write down what you are doing at that moment. Note what you should be doing, if you're not doing it. Write down the activities that did not contribute to your goals (and the length of time each took). Write down any activities you did or are doing that you could eliminate or scale down. Now ask yourself "Are there better or more efficient ways to group or organize some of the activities I did today?" If you analyze your quiz, you should be able to spot some significant areas for improvement. People's perceptions of time spent are generally quite different from the reality of the situation.

- **Be energy conscious.** Observe your personal energy cycle, advises writer Melissa Wahl in the July/August 1992 *Executive Female*. Save nondemanding tasks, such as opening mail, emptying trash, and other routine office or housekeeping chores, for when you're not at your highest mental peak. Every person's body chemistry is different, so tailor your off-peak schedule to fit yours. If you're alert and raring to go in the morning, that's when you should be doing the mentally demanding work of the day in order to make the most of your time.

- **Pad your estimate.** Allocate whatever time you think an activity will take, then add 10 percent.

✓ *Don't procrastinate.*

Procrastination lessens productivity, not only compounding stress but also causing the stressful by-products of guilt, anger, and low self-esteem. About 20 percent of American adults procrastinate enough to suffer personal and/or professional consequences, according to a recent DePaul University study. That percentage threatens to grow, according to business psychologist Harry Levinson, because the worse stress gets, the greater the tendency to procrastinate becomes.

We procrastinate for a whole variety of reasons: fear of success (or failure), fear of separation from a project once it's finished, fear of criticism, fear of authority. The task itself may be complex or too tedious. To help yourself understand why you procrastinate, list and analyze the situations when you do. Are they limited to a particular segment of your life or spread throughout? Are they tasks with no immediate payoffs? Are there immediate consequences that could be tough to handle? Once you've identified the times when you procrastinate, head off your habit by breaking down the task into smaller parts and assigning each a priority and a deadline.

✓ *Live by lists.*

Having a daily written list of what you expect to do will help you become more realistic about your schedule and remind you of tasks you do not want to forget. By listing a task, you also relieve stress by removing the thought from your mind, which helps to lessen mental overload, a common occurrence in stressed people. People who have trouble falling asleep are often told to prepare to-do lists for the next day shortly before bedtime, because listing things helps reduce the tension of a cluttered mind.

Finally, checking off each task you have finished allows you to take note of the day's accomplishments and restores a sense of control and self-esteem, both stress relievers.

✓ *Don't answer to your phone.*

The telephone—one of society's most intrusive stressors—interrupts you from your private time or mid-task and chips away at your sense of control, if you let it. The trick is to master the telephone before it masters you. Here's how: Whether you're in an office or at home, choose a time every day as phone time and let prospective callers know. Except for your designated phone time, refer all calls to a secretary, office mate, answering machine, or voice-mail network. Have your secretary or machine explain that you are busy at the moment but that you will be calling back at a particular time. Then be sure you do—procrastinating on a callback only adds the dread of anticipation until the deed is done.

Take control of your calls. Jot down points you want to make before you dial the number. Decide how long you have to spend on the call and announce this at the outset. ("I have only 10 minutes before I have to be at my next appointment.") Keep a timer by your phone. When the time you've allocated is up, be polite, prompt, and firm. ("I'm going to have to say good-bye now. It's been really nice talking with you.") A psychiatrist who counsels people after stress breakdowns advises his patients to arm themselves with a litany of escape tactics in case there's trouble breaking the connection. ("I have to run—someone's at the door" or "My boss has just asked me to come to her office.")

✔ Become an expert organizer.

Disorganization probably wastes more time and creates more stress than any other single characteristic. But the skill of organization can be learned. Start by thinking about what you want to accomplish in a given time period and determine how to do the task(s) most efficiently. Establish specific times and frequencies for your activities and stick to them. You might, for example, run errands at the drugstore and supermarket only on Thursdays. Make sure you aren't doing things out of habit. Ask yourself why you are doing an activity or following a particular routine. Weigh whether doing it differently—or not doing it at all—would save time or stress.

If paper flow at home or work is overwhelming, try to remove your name from mailing lists. Inquire at the post office, or if you're a credit card holder, exercise the privilege the companies extend to you to remove your name from mailing lists they sell. What paper you must handle, handle only once—to take action or to throw it out. Keep all of your bills in one place and set aside time each week to assemble and pay them. If your office, basement, or closets are such a disorganized mess that you can't get started, consider hiring an organization expert or a cleaning service for a day's visit.

✔ Call a time-out.

Build in some escapes and try some creative time-outs from your stress. Are you a mom who's stressed out at home with the baby? Rotate duties with some other mothers who would also like a day off, creating a "Mother's Day Out" program. If you're a caregiver to an elderly person or a chronically ill loved one, try a variation on the "Day Out" theme. Try also to take advantage of your "wasted" time—the time you're forced to spend standing in line, waiting in the doctor's office, or stopped in traffic—in a creative way. Catch up on pleasure or business reading, make a list, practice relaxation strategies, or just organize your thoughts.

✔ *Allow yourself a margin for the unanticipated.*
Many of life's events are beyond our control. If you allow stress to stretch your inner resources to the limit, you may lack the resilience you need to accommodate unanticipated turns of fortune or misfortune. If you have spent your bank account to the last dollar, you'll face stress when your car needs a new part. If you have a vital 2:00 P.M. appointment that's 30 minutes across town, leaving for it at 1:30 P.M.—without allowing time for traffic or delays—also adds greatly to your stress. (Experts recount one of the simplest techniques to manage the manageable while also preparing for the unforeseen emergency: Keep a full or nearly full tank of gas in your car.)

DIET AND NUTRITION

Believe it or not, what you eat can promote or relieve stress and help or hinder the body in how it handles the physical stress response. To stay healthy and stress-resistant, try these tips.

✓ *Take time out for meals.*
By making your mealtime your oasis from stress, you
can add to your overall health and well-being. Stress puts
a strain on the digestive system by encouraging the over-
production of acids needed in the digestion process.
Stress can also cause malabsorption of nutrients or stomach pain, which occurs when the digestive system is in
spasm.

Eat breakfast sitting in front of your favorite window
or, in warm weather, on an outdoor patio where you can
hear natural sounds. At lunchtime, choose a setting different from the one where you spend the rest of your
stress-filled workday. Let others know that your
mealtimes are off-limits for stressful conversations or
frenetic surroundings. Avoid doing business over every
meal. A power meal with business associates once in a
while won't hurt you, but when it's your daily diet, it
adds to your stress level, stymies your digestive processes, and exacerbates your body's chronic stress response.

Also make a point of eating at regular times, especially when you're trying to combat stress. When you
skip meals, you don't tolerate stress as well because you
lack energy and can't concentrate. Stress and missed
meals can also trigger hypoglycemia, a disorder in which
blood sugar levels are too low. It is characterized by an
increased heart rate, light-headedness or the shakes, and
an anxious or irritable mood. *Alternative Medicine* notes
that many who suffer from hypoglycemia may be ge-
netically predisposed to the disorder.*

---

*Puyallup, Wash.: Future Medicine Publishing, 1994.

A Crash Course in Nutrition

Good nutrition supports cell and tissue reproduction, maintains muscle strength and the skeletal system, and gives your body the fuel it needs, both to endure stress and to keep the immune system in high gear. Understanding the basics of nutrition is a vital part of stress reduction and good health.

The U.S. Department of Agriculture emphasizes a diet rich in grains and complex carbohydrates, fresh vegetables, and fruits. The highest percentage of your day's food should be whole-grain breads, cereals, rice, and pasta (6 to 11 servings), followed by vegetables (3 to 5), fruits (2 to 4), then milk, yogurt, and cheese (2 to 3). Fats (including meats, once the centerpiece of our dinner tables), oils, and sweets should be used sparingly.

The three classes of organic compounds that make up our food are carbohydrates, fats, and proteins. Carbohydrates provide energy and the transport essential for getting vitamins and other nutrients into our bodies. They come in two basic forms: *simple* (glucose, fructose, or galactose, in fruits, sugars, honey, and milk) and *complex* (starches and fiber, in grains, potatoes, pasta, vegetables, and legumes). Fiber, which can be soluble (capable of being dissolved in water) or insoluble, is especially important in times of stress. Insoluble fiber is thought to perform a cleaning function by scraping the walls of the digestive system of carcinogens, cancer-causing agents likely to build up under stress. Studies show that in countries where there is greater intake of foods high in insoluble fiber, there are fewer cases of colon and rectal cancer, and the mortality rates are lower. Soluble fiber slows digestion, improving and regulating the absorption of nutrients into the bloodstream, which helps prevent sudden drops or increases in blood sugar.

Fats have both plant and animal origins. Under normal conditions, the body metabolizes fats into glucose, which it stores until energy is needed. When the body is stressed, metabolism changes to ensure that ready energy is available for the "attack." Glucose is dumped into the bloodstream, and more cortisol and catecholamines (brain chemicals that stimulate the appetite for more fats and simple sugars, other sources of instant energy) are produced. Cortisol makes the body retain fluid, in preparation for a water shortage in the stress emergency, and stimulates a craving for salt.

Proteins provide strength and long-lasting energy and regulate and maintain body growth. They also perform the critical function of bringing into the body its building blocks, the amino acids. These are the natural substances that the body needs in order to formulate body and brain chemicals such as serotonin (the sleep-inducing neurotransmitter whose production is initiated by the amino acid tryptophan) and norepinephrine (the stress hormone launched when we ingest a protein containing the amino acid tyrosine). Most proteins come from animal sources, which are high in fats.

You can treat hypoglycemia by eating a balanced meal that avoids refined carbohydrates (such as white breads and sugars), then getting back on your normal eating schedule. Harvey Ross, M.D., a Los Angeles psychiatrist, recommends a high-protein, low-carbohydrate diet that is broken into five smaller meals, rather than three big meals, a day. Snacks are high in protein. He also has his patients take vitamin supplements.†

✓ *Avoid sugars and fats.*
It's critical to eat well when you're under stress. Unfortunately, that's also the time you probably least feel like eating healthy and are instinctively drawn to comfort foods: a milk shake, a grilled cheese sandwich, a chocolate sundae, meat loaf with gravy. When you're stressed, steer clear of junk foods that are high in simple sugars, such as colas and cupcakes. Simple sugars stimulate the release of epinephrine and intensify the stress reaction while acting as sedatives at a time when you may need to be mentally alert.

Fats may also be guilty of stealing energy you may need at a time of stress. Because they take longer to digest than all other foods and divert blood from the brain and the muscles to aid in digestion, they can enervate you and make you sluggish. Fats can also contribute to heart disease and obesity and complicate the negative effects that stress already has on cardiovascular health.

If you absolutely must indulge yourself to get through a crisis, do it once, but get back on a nutritious diet right away.

---

†*Alternative Medicine.*

✔ **Use stress-reducing foods to your advantage.**
Stress can't be eliminated from your life just by changing your diet, but it is possible to greatly reduce stress if you know which foods influence your state of mind.

If you are stressed out and need a break from your anxiety, try foods low in fat and protein and high in complex carbohydrates for a calming effect, suggests Cooper in his book *Performance Edge*. These foods include cooked whole grains (wheat, oatmeal, buckwheat, or barley) with fruit or sweetener but no milk, low-fat pasta salad with fruit or vegetables, or low-fat, high-grain bread (bagel, muffin, or pita chips) with your favorite fruit preserves.

In Food: *Your Miracle Medicine*, food author Jean Carper suggests calming foods containing the trace element selenium (such as sea-food and grapes) or the mild sedative quercetin (such as onions) as well as foods that act on neurons in the brain to sedate, such as ginger, sugar, and honey.* Foods that stimulate production of serotonin (foods high in folic acid, such as legumes and leafy vegetables) are also calming. Carper's list also includes anise, celery seed, cloves, cumin, fennel, garlic, lime or orange peel, marjoram, parsley, sage, spearmint, and various decaffeinated teas.

However, if you're looking to concentrate your energy to help you get through a stressful day, look for a food that enhances alertness. In Carper's book, neuro-endocrinologist Judith Wurtman, Ph.D., of the Massachusetts Institute of Technology, recommends a low-carbohydrate, high-protein, low-fat meal or snack,

*New York: HarperCollins, 1993.

CONTROLLING ENERGY LEVELS

Eating the right balance of foods can help strengthen your resistance to stress. But did you know that *when* you eat certain foods can also boost or diminish your ability to cope with stress? To get the most from your meals and maximize your resistance to stress, try the combinations below.

- **Breakfast.** Richard Podell, M.D., clinical professor of medicine at the Robert Wood Johnson Medical School, recommends "compact carbohydrates" such as coarse (not instant) oatmeal or all-bran cereal to help keep your blood sugar levels steady.* These densely structured carbohydrates don't break down in the body as quickly as muffins, many breads, and "flaky" cereals, which give your blood sugar an instant boost, then drop you flat in only two to four hours, Podell says. Include, too, a protein (milk, egg, or yogurt) and a citrus juice or fruit. But skip pineapple, watermelon, and raisins, says Podell, since all are high in sugar.
- **Lunch.** To maintain your energy levels through the middle of the day, try a protein for lunch. Neuroendocrinologist Judith Wurtman, Ph.D., of the Massachusetts Institute of Technology, explains that proteins are good at hold-

---

McCall's (August 1994).

ing tyrosine, an amino acid that boosts stress resistance, in your system. Steer clear of complex carbohydrates, such as pasta salad, at lunch unless you eat a protein with them. As we said before, carbohydrates make you feel calm, mellow, and sleepy. While they may provide a calming effect when you're stressed out and ready for a break, they may add to your stress at lunchtime when you're trying to keep your energy up.

- **Dinner.** While eating complex carbohydrates without proteins at lunchtime may diminish your alertness, you may want to put these natural relaxers on your dinner menu. Wurtman notes that just 1.5 ounces of potato, rice, pasta, bread, air-popped popcorn, or low-cal cookie will stimulate the release of serotonin and help calm you at the end of the day.

- **Before bed.** You may remember that the amino acid tyrosine stimulates the release of epinephrine and dopamine, stress hormones that make you more alert. While you may want to eat tyrosine-rich foods during the day if you are stressed and need to be mentally energized, you don't want to make the mistake of eating them near bedtime, when they can prevent a good night's sleep. Tyrosine-rich foods include aged cheeses (blue, Stilton, Parmesan), soft cheeses (mozzarella, Swiss, feta), red wine, yogurt, sour cream, cured and processed meats and fish, yeast products, eggplant, potatoes, spinach, and tomatoes.

making sure you start with the protein. Devoting 5 to 10 percent of a meal to protein will offset the sedating effects of carbohydrates and help ward off a serotonin buildup, which makes us mentally sluggish. Such low-carbohydrate, high-protein foods include meat or cheese sauce on pasta, tuna on a roll, low-fat seafood (plain shrimp or tuna in water), turkey breast, skim milk, or low-fat yogurt. Don't forget fruits and nuts: These contain high levels of the trace mineral boron, which affects the electrical activity of the brain, says Carper. You'll need only an ounce or two of such a snack to get an alertness effect.

✔ Avoid the foods that set off stress pain.

When you're operating under stress, pamper your body by avoiding foods that don't agree with you. Stress makes the digestive system work erratically and over-time, increasing the levels of gastric acid churning in the stomach. So if you have a condition such as colitis, ir-ritable bowel syndrome, or hiatal hernia, stay away from highly spiced or greasy foods.

Stress also intensifies allergic reactions, such as hives and difficulty breathing, so try to avoid your particular trigger foods and substances. And since stress may also aggravate migraine headaches, those prone should stay away from foods containing the amino acid tyrosine—aged cheeses, red wine, and cured meats among them. Those with hypoglycemia should take extra care to avoid sugary foods, and those who have difficulty tolerating lactose would be wise to exclude all milk and whey-containing foods in periods of stress.

Avoid caffeine as well. Caffeine, the psychoactive "natural upper" that's found in coffee, many teas, and a variety of soft drinks as well as in chocolate and selected other foods, acts in the body like a shot of epinephrine, increasing the heart rate, blood pressure, and heart oxygen levels. Duke University research found higher amounts of the hormones related to stress in the bodies of coffee drinkers than in those who drank a placebo (inactive substance).

✔ *Watch out for stress-triggered compulsions.*

Highly stressful situations often trigger reactions in the form of destructive habits or urges. When they are stressed, some people eat more, drink more, smoke or smoke more, double up on their caffeine intake, go on impulsive shopping sprees, or engage in compulsive sex. Giving in to these impulses makes them feel tranquil and helps them get through their stress. Too often in the end, however, guilt about the excessive behavior is added to the original stressful situation, compounding stress rather than eliminating it.

Overeating and compulsive eating typically affect those who haven't learned to handle stress or how to express anxiety and tension orally. If overeating (or any compulsive behavior) is your pattern when you're feeling stressed, you may need to join a support group or seek professional counseling to help you change your behavior. (Chapter 3 will say more about therapy.) If you don't consider yourself an addictive eater but you tend to snack constantly when stress gets bad, anticipate your stressful moments by stocking the refrigerator with healthy, low-calorie foods: carrot and celery sticks, apples, flavored rice cakes, low-fat flavored yogurt, bottled water (beware of flavored waters, which are often sweetened), and herbal teas.

Those susceptible to destructive urges when stressed need to be vigilant about avoiding the behavior as well as the stressful situations that may invite a trigger reaction. Participants in 12-step recovery programs such as Alcoholics Anonymous are taught that they're most likely to give into destructive urges when they are hungry, angry, lonely, or tired, situations remembered by the acronym HALT.

VITAMIN, MINERAL, AND HERBAL THERAPY

Use these natural ingredients in your diet to give yourself an edge against stress.

✔ *Replace the vitamins and minerals that stress depletes.*
Signs of vitamin depletion can include depression, anxiety, gastric upset, and insomnia, which, of course, are also symptoms of too much stress.

James F. Balch, M.D., author of *Prescription for Nutritional Healing*, suggests making certain your daily multivitamin has the following ingredients and amounts if you're under stress.* It's a good idea to check with your doctor before you begin any vitamin, mineral, or herbal therapy. Keep in mind that many of these recommendations are higher than the *minimum* daily requirements, and that mega-dosing—adding units beyond the totals suggested here—can be dangerous to your health.

---

*Garden City Park, N.Y.: Avery, 1990.

• **Vitamin A:** 15,000 (10,000 for pregnant women) international units daily. This vitamin helps adrenal gland function and promotes healthy growth of epithelial cells, including those lining the blood vessels. *Food sources*: cod-liver oil, beef, liver, oysters, butter, whole milk, and orange and green leafy vegetables such as carrots, sweet potatoes, mangoes, spinach, turnip greens, and romaine lettuce.

• **Vitamin B-complex:** 100 milligrams daily. These vitamins help the nervous system function, reduce anxiety and immune system damage, and improve brain function. Within the B-complex family, 100 milligrams of pantothenic acid (B_5) can be used three times a day in heavy stress periods. Also include 50 milligrams daily of pyridoxine (B_6), which influences neurotransmitters and helps convert tryptophan to serotonin. *Food sources*: chicken, fish, pork, eggs, brown rice, soybeans, and oats.

• **Vitamin C:** 3,000 to 10,000 milligrams daily. A powerful antioxidant (a molecule that cleans your system of cancer-causing free radicals), vitamin C boosts the immune system and is needed to produce connective tissue, which helps maintain the structure of tissues, including blood vessels. Vitamin C reduces some allergic responses and helps offset the depletion of adrenal gland hormones caused by stress. *Food sources*: citrus fruits and their juices, red bell peppers, black currants, guava, strawberries, broccoli, brussels sprouts, and papaya.

• **Vitamin E:** 400 international units. Vitamin E is the strongest antioxidant and works with vitamin C and selenium to help strengthen the immune system, fight heart disease, promote healthy nerve function, and minimize the damage to muscles caused by free radicals. *Food sources*: hazelnut oil, wheat germ oil, sunflower oil, almond oil, wheat germ, mayonnaise, whole-grain cereals, eggs, and fortified cereals.

• **Calcium:** 2,000 milligrams daily. Calcium relaxes muscles, builds bone, reduces intestinal irritation, and lowers blood pressure. *Food sources*: milk and dairy products, kale, turnip greens, canned salmon, sardines with bones, and soybeans.

• **Magnesium:** 1,000 milligrams daily. Stress researcher Leon Chaitow, D.O., in *Stress*, notes that this element is vital for nerve conditioning, muscle contraction, and transmission of impulses through the nervous system. It works in the production of energy from sugar and reacts with calcium to affect functions such as heartbeat. Low intakes of magnesium are associated with high blood pressure and heart disease. *Food sources*: whole grains, nuts, avocados, beans, and dark green leafy vegetables.

• **Potassium:** Potassium is especially needed during stress because it promotes adrenal gland functioning. It also helps muscle contraction, nerve conduction, heartbeat regulation, and energy production. It interacts with sodium to regulate the body's fluid balance and can have an effect in lowering blood pressure. Though Balch does not recommend a specific amount, the National Research Council suggests 1,600 to 2,000 milligrams daily. *Food sources*: fruits, especially bananas; vegetables and their juices; baked potatoes, especially the skins; yams; prunes; raisins; shellfish; and beans.

• **Selenium:** 70 micrograms for men, 55 micrograms for women. Selenium is a trace mineral with antioxidant properties that helps prevent some cancers and heart disease (it prevents the buildup of fats in arteries and damage to blood vessel walls). It also boosts the immune system. *Food sources*: broccoli, celery, cucumbers, onions, garlic, radishes, brewer's yeast, grains, fish, and organ meats.

- **Zinc:** 50 milligrams. This essential element is involved in the production of more than 200 body enzymes. It helps heal wounds, promotes healthy skin, and boosts immune function. It is available as a zinc gluconate lozenge. *Food sources*: oysters, beef, pork and beef liver, lamb, crab, and wheat germ.

✔ *Give your vitamins a boost.*
Phytochemicals, a newly discovered class of natural compounds found in various fruits and vegetables but not in supplements, give the vitamins they accompany a supercharge. "Phytos" that pack a big wallop include the following:

- **Sulforaphane,** found in cruciferous vegetables (broccoli, cabbage, brussels sprouts), helps block tumors.
- **Allylic sulfides,** found in garlic and onions, strengthen the immune system, fight chronic conditions such as stomach cancer, and may help to lower blood pressure when eaten regularly.
- **Flavonoids** (or bioflavonoids), found in green plants, just under the skin of citrus fruits, and in some berries, enhance vitamin C absorption.

Bottom line: If given the choice between taking an ascorbic acid (vitamin C) pill and eating a freshly peeled orange, go for the orange every time. (And be sure to include some of the white part of the peel just under the skin.)

✓ *Try herbals and botanicals to help relieve stress.*
Teas made from plants with calming properties have
been used for centuries to abate stress. Several principal
herbals stand out for their calming, sedating, tranquiliz-
ing qualities

- **Chamomile.** Its dried flowers steeped as tea have
  anti-inflammatory, relaxant, and antispasmodic
  properties and are said to promote relaxation, decrease stress levels, and settle the stomach. Be cau-
  tious of this herbal if you suffer from hay fever or
  other plant allergies, as chamomile can trigger a
  serious reaction.
- **Valerian.** Its root extract makes a tea that, for most
  people, is a natural tranquilizer, sedative, and
  calmative that doesn't leave a groggy hangover, if
  taken properly. Valerian is an active ingredient of
  nonprescription sleep aids, here and in Europe. Valerian has two problems: The root's intensity varies
  by plant, according to the September/October 1995
  Natural Health, which results in nonuniform product strengths, and it smells terrible. To avoid the
  odor, try capsules of dried valerian root, or sweeten
  the tea with honey or flavor it with lemon. For 5
  percent of the population, valerian is a stimulant
  that increases anxiety, so watch for side effects.
- **Passionflower.** As with chamomile, its tea is made
  from pulverized flowers. It is recommended for
  chronic worriers or those with overbusy minds.
- **Catnip.** For all but cats, its dried flowers and
  leaves act as a sedative when taken as tea before
  bed; antispasmodic properties soothe the stomach.

USING HERBALS WISELY

Even though most people in the United States use herbals as supplements, they should still be treated as drugs. Herbals and other natural remedies were humankind's original drugs (the word *drug* comes from the German *droge*, meaning "to dry," acknowledgment of the preparation process for herbals and botanicals).

Herbals are not regulated by the Food and Drug Administration, but for the past few years that oversight agency has published a list of herbals it considers unsafe. Research any herbals you plan to take, then check with your medical practitioner before starting any herbal regimen. Herbals and prescribed medicines do occasionally interact. Similarly, megadosing can be dangerous. And for some, notably those with allergies or heart disease, some herbals can be lethal. Certain herbs can also cause miscarriage in pregnant women. Herbalists, like their medical counterparts, recommend identifying underlying causes of stress rather than relying on herbal preparations for a long period of time to alleviate the symptoms of stress.

Most recipes for herbal tea call for two teaspoons of the root powder or pulverized leaf/flower, allowed to steep for 10 to 15 minutes in very hot, not boiling, water. (Be sure to check each product for specific directions.)

Other herbals traditionally mentioned for counteracting stress include hops, lady's slipper, pau d'arco, rose hips, rosemary, melissa, Siberian and American ginseng, and skullcap.

EXERCISE

To work away your tension and fortify yourself against the negative physical effects of stress, try these tips.

✔ *Squeeze something.*
When you're stressed, squeezing something, such as those squishy, semimalleable hand exercisers, often triggers relaxation and a release of the body's fight-or-flight response. You don't even need to follow a specific set of exercises or squeeze rhythmically—it's the action of squeezing that does the trick.

In prehistoric times, this emergency alert was universally answered with a physical response. In modern times, which are filled with psychological stressors, few fight-or-flight responses demand immediate physical solutions, so the muscles stay "on the ready." The big squeeze helps satisfy that lingering physical urge.

✔ *Hang loose.*
Get into the habit of regularly checking and loosening your body's tense spots. This "rag doll" exercise will make you aware of how stress is being felt in your body and will help loosen tight muscles and reduce your stress.

First, relax tight jaw muscles by assuming a resting-jaw position: upper and lower teeth slightly apart, tongue touching neither. Then relax your hands, making sure your fingers are not flexed. And pay attention to your shoulders: If they're slouched forward or scrunched tightly together, loosen them.

Every hour stand up and let your shoulders drop and

your arms and hands dangle. Drop your chin to your chest and roll your head from shoulder to shoulder. Shake your dangling hands a few times.

✓ *Try aerobic exercise.*

Aerobic exercise—sustained, regular exercise that builds lung capacity, increases cardiovascular health, and burns body fat—also reduces stress. After 10 to 20 minutes of intense exercise, the brain releases epinephrine and endorphins, tension-lowering chemicals, into the system. Epinephrine is the stress hormone that gives us a surge of energy to help sustain activity while improving blood circulation, which cleans the cells of toxins and debilitating lactic acid that accrue when we're stressed and inactive. However, it does not increase stress because it is offset by endorphins, the stress-fighting chemicals that provide a sense of well-being.

Before you begin a regimen, consult a professional trainer or your doctor to determine the exercise program that's best for you, and be sure to pick an exercise you like. Two notes of caution: First, don't aim to achieve a level of exercise that is unrealistic. As writer Daryn Eller notes in the June 6, 1995, *Redbook*, unrealistic expectations are apt to make you feel guilty when you fall short, undoing all the good. Second, don't overdo: Too much exercise can strain the heart and push your stress level higher.

You may also try sex to get your heart rate up. Research has shown that sexual stimulation releases not only positive endorphins but also, in women, the sex hormones progesterone and estrogen. All these hormones help make us feel mellow and less sensitive to pain (and stress). And once the sexual drive is satisfied,

STRESS AND YOUR MUSCLES

Not even the body's muscular system escapes damage from stress. Under prolonged stress, many of our muscle cells are starved in two ways. Stress causes shallow breathing, so we take in less fresh oxygen than healthy cells require. Instead of nourishing all the muscles, the nutrient- and oxygen-carrying blood is being directed to the organs and muscles most needed for the stress response. In addition, cellular waste in the form of lactic acid, a major nerve irritant, is not being removed through the veins. The result is a muscle spasm, a painful involuntary contraction that occurs when muscles are exhausted and depleted of nutrients. Chronically stressed muscles eventually shorten and lose their elasticity, creating ideal conditions for serious muscle injury.

Back pain and minor back injuries are common results of this relationship between muscles and stress. In a New York University and Columbia University study of more than 5,000 cases of back pain, 81 percent were related to muscle problems—problems that are often triggered, if not caused, by stress. However, exercise and stress management can help keep muscles in top shape.

the body's natural reaction is total relaxation, certainly an antidote to stress.

✓ Take a walk.

Walking is a natural stress buster, regardless of pace. At California State University, researchers found that the

stimulation of just a 10-minute walk is enough to increase energy, alter mood, and effect a positive outlook
for up to two hours. A University of Massachusetts Center for Health and Fitness study, highlighted in *The Wellness Encgclopedia*, found that a brisk 40-minute walk
drops anxiety levels by an average of 14 percent.

✔ Get into the swim of relaxation.

For centuries, water has been known for its healing properties. Swimming can relieve muscle tension and joint
stiffness caused by stress. (Swimming is especially helpful to those suffering from arthritis or any condition that
limits joint or limb movement.) Water helps support
your body, permitting your muscles a time-out from
maintaining stress-effected poor posture. Jenny Sutcliffe,
author of *The Complete Book of Relaxation Techniques*,
suggests that you swim hard to rid yourself of aggression
or "laze along" to banish fatigue and anxiety.* Or, says
Sutcliffe, try floating with your eyes closed as you imagine all the tension draining out of your body and into
the water.

✔ Don't let stress give you a pain in the neck.

In times of stress, we tend to elevate—or pull together—
our shoulders in a tense, rigid formation without realizing it. This musculoskeletal abuse can lead to painful
damage such as a pinched neck nerve or a muscle spasm,
which may later trigger pain that radiates down an arm
and even into the hand.

A quick exercise to relax neck and shoulder muscles,
found in Lawrence Galton's *Coping With Executive*

---

*Allentown, Pa.: People's Medical Society, 1994.

Stress, consists of elevating your shoulders, shaking them back down, and then, at a moderate speed, wiggling your shoulders up and around to create an "uneven" motion that affects both shoulders at once.† Drop your head and roll it to the right, then to the left, trying to touch each ear to the shoulder. All of these help stretch and relax muscles. (If you do any of these and experience pain, stop immediately and consult a doctor.)

Charleston, South Carolina, sports physician Anthony C. Ross, D.C., believes toning and strengthening the deeper muscle groups that support the cervical spine can reduce neck problems. He suggests you stand with your shoulder against a wall and place a 10-inch inflatable rubber ball between your head (just above your right ear) and the wall. While standing straight, push against the ball with your head until the ball "gives." Push from the neck, *not* from below the shoulders. Repeat 10 times, then do the same with the other side of the head. Then place the ball between your forehead and the wall for 10 reps. Finally, stand with the ball behind your lower back, holding the ball against the wall. Squat slowly, allowing the ball to "migrate" up your spine, then rise again to a standing position, allowing the ball to move vertically down the length of the spine.

✔ *Learn and maintain good, antistress posture.*
Hunching your shoulders, a typical "stress posture," throws off your whole system of balance, resulting in the musculoskeletal damage and accompanying problems we mentioned earlier. Maintaining good posture is a learned skill. Bess Mensendieck, M.D., a Dutch

---

†New York: McGraw Hill, 1983.

sculptor-turned-physician, established criteria for good standing posture that are now known as the Mensendieck Technique, which is widely taught throughout Europe:*

- Set your feet parallel, exactly below the hip joints, with the balls of the feet two inches apart, the toes straight ahead, and the heels straight back.
- Raise your pelvis by tucking the buttocks firmly together and slightly under.
- Contract your abdominal muscles firmly upward while maintaining a tall stance.
- Draw your shoulder blades toward the spinal column and downward (allowing them to "squeeze" the vertebrae in midback), which brings the sternum (breastbone) into its diagonally forward-up position.
- Extend your neck upward to your crown, letting your head rest, well poised, on your spine. (Your arms will automatically come precisely alongside your body.)
- Equally distribute your weight over your heels and the bases of your big toes.

✓ *Work your jaw.*
Similar to the stress posture, the human jaw can be considered a barometer of stress. When we are tense, we often clench our jaws without realizing it. Some of us clench and grind our teeth in sleep until, in worst cases, the teeth become worn and cracked and the jaw aches perpetually. A professor at Tufts University School of Dental Medicine, mentioned in the December 4, 1995,

---

Your Posture and Your Pains. Anchor, 1973.

issue of *Newsweek*, has estimated that as much as 20 percent of the population grinds its teeth destructively Temporomandibular joint disorder occurs after chronic clenching and triggers migraines, jaw dislocation, tooth damage, and neck and head muscle pain.

To rescue a sore jaw and your teeth from the pressures created by too much stress, become conscious of your jaw. Are you clenching it now? Do you clench at night or when stress is at its worst? Try to relax your jaw by letting it go slack, touching your lips together but keeping a space between your upper and lower teeth. Teach yourself to hold your tongue in a position that is not touching your teeth. (It's almost impossible to clench if you can do this.) Work out your worries before bed, if you grind at night. If that doesn't work, consider getting a night-guard retainer from your dentist to preserve your teeth.

✓ Exercise on the job.

If you spend most of your days at a desk, phone, or computer, you can try these exercises to help relieve stress and possibly prevent damaging repetitive motion injuries:

- Do periodic exercises with your hands. Massage them inside and out with your thumbs and fingers. Gently bend your wrists back and forth. Make a fist and open the hand a few times.
- Get up at least once an hour, even if it's just to move around your workstation and stretch.
- At least hourly, shift your eyes away from the monitor to focus on a distant object. Eye muscles

have to work harder to focus on close objects such
as a monitor.

- Get a headset instead of cradling your phone between your ear and your shoulder.

SELF-CARE

Take your stress prevention efforts one step further with
these easy-to-learn self-care methods.

✓ *Try sunlight therapy.*

Stressed people need to make an extra effort to take in
adequate natural light every day. A landmark 1980 study
cited in Weiner and Brown's *Office Biology* showed that
limited-spectrum artificial lighting—the kind often used
in offices and schools—actually elevates stress hormone
levels.

The body uses sunlight and full-spectrum light to syn-
thesize vitamin D, which helps the body absorb calcium
and keep blood pressure low—increasing health and
lowering stress. Natural light also regulates the pineal
gland, which oversees many of the body's rhythms.
Without natural light, the gland becomes desensitized,
throwing your already stressed body into worse shape.

When suffering from acute stress, your tendency may
be to burrow into your office or home. Try instead to be
outdoors for at least 30 minutes (preferably an hour) in
the brightest sunlight of the day, which is early morning.
Investigate adding a set of full-spectrum fluorescent
lights to a room in your home or office. Or your health-
care provider (or local lighting distributor) may be able
to tell you where to find full-spectrum light boxes, which
are more portable. Even though not all doctors agree

about the extent to which light therapy relieves stress, they agree that it does help and that sunlight is always preferable to indoor facsimiles.

✔ *Enjoy spa treatment.*

What could be more relaxing than an all-natural facial, an acupressure massage, or a session in a sauna? Of course, not all spas restrict their treatments to pampering: Increasingly, you'll find instruction on stress management, good nutrition, and relaxation techniques, squeezed in between the early morning hike, the late morning workout, and the low-calorie lunch. There are spas to suit every schedule and bank account, from one-day quickies to a full week with the works. (Find one in *The Spa Finder*, an annual publication of about 200 pages that lists, describes, and shows photos of hundreds of spas. It is available for a small charge by calling 800-255-7727.)

If time or money precludes a trip to the spa, fashion one in your own home. The March/April 1995 *Natural Health* magazine suggests you set the spa activities in advance: Lay out all necessary oils, facial rubs, and other balms and lotions and select favorite relaxing music. When your personal spa opens for business, make sure it's understood by housemates that it's off-limits for a couple of hours and divert phone calls to your answering machine.

✔ *Try these relaxation strategies.*

Reaching a state of true, deep relaxation—when your muscles are loose, your heart rate is slower, your breathing is deep, and your mind is clear—requires learned skills and practice. There are many ways to relax. To reduce stress, explore some of the methods described in the chart to find one that suits you. For information on complementary medicine, some forms of which can be used as self-care (for example, yoga and tai chi), see Chapter 3.

Set definite times during your day to relax. Try scheduling 10- to 15-minute sessions at least three times daily—morning, midday, and evening. You'll need a quiet place—away from the phone, radio, television, and other interruptions—that you can have to yourself, even if you have to put a sign on the door so that others will know to keep out. And remember that relaxing doesn't mean doing nothing or being bored. One study that focused on the benefits of true relaxation showed that endorphins—the feel-good hormones—are released into the body during a state of relaxation, but not during one of boredom or just plain inactivity.

MIND/BODY STRATEGIES FOR ACHIEVING THE RELAXATION RESPONSE

	DEFINITION	PROCEDURE	INTENDED RESULT(S)
THE RELAXATION RESPONSE	A natural state of self-induced relaxation, introduced by Herbert Benson, M.D. In the relaxation response, conscious (stress-causing) thoughts are blocked by using a variety of strategies that employ four elements: (1) a mental device (such as an object or a "mantra," a one-syllable word) on which to focus to enhance concentration; (2) a passive attitude; (3) a comfortable, relaxed position; (4) a quiet environment. The relaxation response results in reduced tension, increased alpha (relaxed) brain waves, lower heart and breathing rates, slower metabolism, and decreased digestive acid secretion.		
STRATEGY	**DEFINITION**	**PROCEDURE**	**INTENDED RESULT(S)**
DEEP BREATHING	Slow, rhythmic breathing with deep inhalation and exhalation. Concentration on breathing allows you to put aside conscious stress and focus on relaxation. It is often used in combination with other strategies.	Stand or sit straight. Slowly inhale and let the abdomen and ribs expand up and out. Exhale from the abdomen, then the chest. Your shoulders should not move toward your ears while inhaling.	Increased oxygen volume refreshes cells and purges cellular waste. The slow rhythm aids relaxation.

PROGRESSIVE MUSCLE RELAXATION	Systematic contracting and relaxing of the muscles. Progressive relaxation breaks tense-mind/tense-muscle syndrome by teaching recognition of physical stress.	Assume a comfortable position, close your eyes, and practice deep breathing. Systematically tense and relax each muscle in order from the toes to the head. Practice for 10 to 20 minutes twice daily (but not while digesting food).	Alternating muscle tension and release helps develop awareness of the physical effects of stress. Practice allows you to relax at will.
VISUALIZATION THERAPY Reframing, internal or guided imagery, safe-haven therapy	A change in perception or the visualization of a pleasurable situation that serves as a mental way to combat stress.	Close your eyes and envision controlling a stressor. Assign it a definition (red blobs may signify anxiety), then change your perception (imagine the blobs stuffed into a bottle, then picture yourself tossing it into the garbage). Or imagine a pleasant, soothing object, scene, or event.	Visualization promotes deep relaxation, which causes a release of serotonin, a calming hormone that alleviates muscle tension and promotes healing.

STRATEGY	DEFINITION	PROCEDURE	INTENDED RESULT(S)
MEDITATION Transcendental meditation, self-hypnosis	Concentration on one object while ignoring external stimuli to promote relaxation. (This was the inspiration for Benson's relaxation response.)	Sit or lie comfortably, close your eyes, and silently repeat a one-syllable word (or mantra) continuously. Focus on the word to prevent distraction. Practice for 10 to 20 minutes twice a day or whenever stressed.	Oxygen consumption decreases 10 to 20 percent. Heartbeat, breathing, and metabolism slow, and blood pressure drops.
MINDFULNESS Present living, attention-to-life training	Concentration on present, tangible situations to purge from the mind stressful, anxiety-producing thoughts about the past or future.	Focus on the physical attributes of objects around you (the color of the walls or the shape of a lamp) to keep your mind from wandering. This is often used to maximize the relaxing effects of other strategies.	The mind is calmed and distracted from intangible, stressful thoughts.

AROMATHERAPY	Inhalation or application of fragrant essential oils extracted from plants and flowers to promote relaxation, healing, and sleep.	In a stress-free setting, bathe in warm water containing a blend of oils such as marjoram, lavender, geranium, chamomile, sandalwood, lily of the valley, rose, and apple spice. Fragrances can also be imparted through scented candles, perfumes, skin lotions, and massage oils.	Fragrances prompt olfactory receptors to signal the portion of the brain that control emotions and memories, prompting a release of calming hormones and an increase in alpha and theta (calming) brain waves.
HYDROTHERAPY	Use of water to change body temperature (hydrothermal therapy) and promote relaxation. It includes swimming, bathing, showering, and using a whirlpool or sauna. Substances such as herbs may also be added to the water (hydrochemical therapy) to aid relaxation.	A natural bath (92° to 96°F) for one-half hour to two hours sedates. A warm or hot bath (98° to 104°F) for 5 to 15 minutes relieves muscle tension. A 30-minutes soak before bed promotes sleep. Herbal baths affect muscles and blood flow.	Warm water induces the release of endorphins and serotonin and stimulates healing. Warm or hot water dilates blood vessels, while cold constricts them. Both help improve circulation, enhancing relaxation. Buoyancy takes pressure off taut muscles.

STRATEGY	DEFINITION	PROCEDURE	INTENDED RESULT(S)
MUSIC THERAPY	Use of music to relax and soothe. It can be used alone or in combination with other strategies.	Play flowing, relaxing music, preferably with a rhythm of one beat per second. Listen in a comfortable position with eyes closed, using headphones if necessary. Imagine that the music is water flowing around you, washing away your tension.	Soothing music affects the right hemisphere of the brain (the seat of emotion), blocking negative and stressful thoughts. Blood pressure drops, heart and breathing rates slow, and endorphins and serotonin are released. Muscle tension decreases.
AUTOGENIC THERAPY OR TRAINING Self-hypnosis	A progression of specific mental commands given to oneself so as to enter a light hypnotic trance, essentially the same state of total relaxation achieved during sleep.	In a reclining position with your eyes closed, repeat commands ("My legs and arms are heavy," "My heart is steady and calm," and so on) until you believe each state is achieved or until a progression through the entire muscle system is reached. Practice in three 20- to 30-minute sessions weekly.	Healing mechanisms work more efficiently during hypnosis. There are physical, psychological, and emotional benefits. With practice, it's possible to induce this state using only a few commands.

BIOFEEDBACK	Consciously controlling involuntary body functions by concentrating to change physical conditions. It is taught by using electronic monitoring of the body's responses.	Muscular tension is measured through electrodes attached to the body. When you are tense, the monitor emits high-pitched sounds. As you relax, the pitch becomes lower.	Concentration can result in the slowing of breathing and heart rate, a change in body temperature, and the release of muscle tension.

Sources: Herbert Benson, M.D., *The Relaxation Response;* Leon Chaitow, D. O., *Stress; Diabetes Forecast;* Robert S. Eliot, M.D., *From Stress to Strength;* John Feltman, et al., *The Prevention How-To Dictionary of Healing Remedies and Techniques;* Lawrence Galton, *Coping With Executive Stress;* Charles B. Inlander and Cynthia K. Moran, *67 Ways to Good Sleep;* Andrew E. Slaby, M.D., Ph.D., M.PH., "Sixty Ways to Make Stress Work for You." *Psychiatry Letter;* Jenny Sutcliffe, *The Complete Book of Relaxation Techniques,* University of California, Berkeley, *The Wellness Encyclopedia;* Laurel Vukovic, "Breathe Deeply . . . and Relax," *Natural Health.*

3

TIPS FOR TREATING STRESS

Regardless of how well you try to manage stress, there might be times when stress gets the better of you. You feel overwhelmed instead of challenged, as well as burned out, powerless, sad, frightened, vulnerable, irrational, and just plain numb. If so, you—along with as much as 68 percent of the adult population—are exhibiting stress symptoms.

This chapter is devoted to tips on the treatment of stress and includes quick tips you can try immediately, as a kind of "stress first aid," as well as advice on medical and complementary treatments and how to seek outside help.

TRADITIONAL MEDICAL INTERVENTION

✓ *Start with a checkup.*
Fatigue, headaches, asthma, a racing heart, nausea or diarrhea, insomnia, effusive sweating, and allergic reactions are all symptoms of stress, but they may mask

those of an underlying disorder or signal the presence of any one of a variety of medical conditions.

Don't mistake depression, a psychological condition that requires professional intervention, for stress, even though they are closely related. Some stress symptoms—inability to sleep through the night, lingering exhaustion, frustration, fear, and continual feelings of sadness or powerlessness—may indicate depression. Various behavioral changes, such as drinking or smoking more than usual, crying more, gaining weight due to atypical, frequent eating urges, and increasing the use of drugs, can also signal depression. (We have more to say about stress-related depression on the next page.)

David S. Bell, M.D., in his book *Chronic Fatigue*, recommends your exam cover at least the following: the American Cancer Society's full cancer screening tests; a complete blood count to detect chronic infection or anemia; a sedimentation rate test, another blood test that screens for a variety of medical abnormalities; tests of routine chemistries to rule out thyroid conditions or problems triggered by arthritis; and a chest x-ray.* Depending on what symptoms you report, your doctor may choose to do other tests as well and may even refer you to a specialist for further testing or treatment, especially if stress is taking a toll on a particular bodily system.

You'll also want to be sure your stress symptoms aren't caused by drug interactions. Mixing medications—including prescriptive drugs, over-the-counter (OTC) medications, and herbal preparations—without first checking for known interactions can, at best, cancel out any benefits the drugs are intended to give and, at worst,

---

*Emmaus, Pa.: Rodale, 1993.

be lethal. List all medications you are currently taking (including all herbals, OTC and prescriptive medications, vitamins, and minerals) as well as their amounts and frequencies and review the list with your medical practitioner. Some medications may be unnecessary or may be replaced by less reactive drugs.

If you have ruled out other medical conditions and are ready to enlist a doctor in your fight against stress, start with your primary care practitioner. Depending on the severity of your complaint, your doctor may recommend some form of mental health counseling or perhaps drug therapy. If you prefer not to start solely with antianxiety medication, tell your doctor and together you can investigate alternatives. If you do start with drug therapy, chart your progress and return to your doctor if you don't notice marked improvement in the time frame indicated.

✓ Learn the distinctions of three serious stress-related conditions.

Even though *burnout, depression,* and *breakdown* are terms sometimes used interchangeably, each condition is distinctive. Here's a primer:

- **Burnout** has recognizable symptoms and results from prolonged stress, says Donald E. Rosen, M.D., a psychiatrist who directs the Professionals in Crisis program at the Menninger Clinic in Topeka, Kansas: "Victims are lethargic, feel empty, and are no longer able to take satisfaction in what they once enjoyed. They have a deep questioning of the value of the tasks they perform."* Fatigue

---

*Fortune (July 25, 1994).

is an important indicator, because burnout generally occurs at the third and most extreme point (exhaustion) of Selye's general adaptation syndrome (see page 3). Extreme burnout, say *Office Biology* authors Edith Weiner and Arnold Brown, is marked by alienation, an indifference to daily activities, and a desire to get away and go to sleep.†
Burnout can be relieved through relaxation techniques (see the chart on page 66–71), improved time management, a healthy diet and exercise routine, and modifications to eliminate, or at least reduce, noise and interruptions. Sometimes time off or time out from the stressful situation is a must. Lack of improvement after self-care probably indicates the need for intervention, either by your primary care physician or by a professional counselor.

- **Depression** has different forms and ranges from mild dysthymia, in which a person simply is irritable and feels bad most of the time, to clinical depression, the umbrella term that indicates severe and long-term symptoms that require treatment, possibly even drug therapy. Depression is a syndrome, or a collection of signs and symptoms. According to the American Psychiatric Association, to be clinically depressed, a person must have at least five of the following symptoms (including the first two) for at least a two-week period (a normal reaction to a recent major trauma, such as the death of a loved one, should not be considered a symptom):

---

†New York: MasterMedia, 1994.

✓ continually depressed mood
✓ markedly diminished pleasure in daily activities
✓ significant weight loss or loss of appetite
✓ insomnia or too much sleep daily
✓ abnormal speeding up or slowing down of one's activities and mental processes
✓ daily fatigue or loss of energy
✓ feelings of worthlessness or inappropriate guilt
✓ diminished ability to think, concentrate, or make decisions
✓ recurrent thoughts of suicide or death

• **Breakdown**, or stress breakdown, results when a person's ability to cope with the ordinary demands of life is severely damaged by stress. Early warnings include unrelenting exhaustion, irritability, a trapped feeling, and fear, fatigue, and frustration.

Symptoms of breakdown are much more severe than those of stress, explains psychiatrist Michael Epstein, M.D., coauthor of *Falling Apart*.* Although most people who suffer stress breakdowns recover, Epstein says, they are often left with a permanent vulnerability to stress: After a breakdown, unlike after a period of less severe stress, stress symptoms and feelings of powerlessness persist. Stress breakdowns may follow untreated burnout and may accompany depression.

In *Falling Apart*, Epstein explains that self-care techniques for stress do not necessarily work with

---

*Sebastopol, Calif.: CRCS, 1992.

breakdown and may even make the situation worse: "Doctors liken it to treating a fractured leg as though it were a strain." Instead, all breakdowns need intervention—early intervention is best—and almost always call for psychotherapy combined with antidepressant medication. And unlike burn-out and most depression, recovery almost always requires leave from work and family responsibility until the situation improves.

✔ *Review your insurance coverage for stress-related conditions.*
Mental health problems emanating from job-related stress constitute a huge chunk of American health care, affecting one in four of us at an annual cost of $200 billion. Scrutinize your health insurance information or call your benefits manager, if you're employed or retired, to find out what your policy covers for stress-related conditions, who offers stress management treatment in your network, and what referrals you need to access it. By being prepared, you'll receive the best treatment for stress.

National media reports in the *New York Times* and the *Wall Street Journal* have warned that many managed care groups are favoring reduced benefits for psychotherapy (or "talk therapy") while emphasizing more economical drug treatments for stress reduction. Managed care officials point to years of excessive psychotherapy costs, while psychotherapists and many medical doctors cite the arguably better and longer-lasting results that occur when stress is treated using a combination of both drug and talk therapies. To date, the managed care entities appear to be winning by limiting the number of psychiatric visits for which a patient can be reimbursed. Where your own policy's coverage is concerned, be a strong advocate.

✓ *Get psychotherapeutic counseling, especially if your stress seems uncontrollable or you suspect depression.*

Psychotherapy is a form of counseling intended to help a person resolve and learn to manage the emotional issues causing mental and physical anxiety. Its goal, other than to relieve current stress, is to teach a person how to express anger and conflict in appropriate ways so that he or she can function more effectively.

Psychotherapeutic counseling is done with a psychiatrist, a specialist trained in mental illness who has a medical degree (doctor of medicine [M.D.] or doctor of osteopathy [D.O.]) and who may prescribe medicine. A psychiatrist must be licensed by the state to practice. Board certification—held by only one in three psychiatrists—is probably not as much of an indicator of skill as are additional training and membership in psychotherapy and/or psychoanalytic associations.

Unless you suspect you suffer from depression, psychotherapy is probably not a wise choice until you have had a full medical exam, as recommended at the start of this chapter. However, once you've ruled out a medical origin of your anxiety and tried some self-help measures such as the ones in Chapter 2 for at least several weeks (the time it takes your body to adjust to new routines), you may consider psychotherapy as the next step on the road to stress control.

Regardless of the form or orientation of counseling used, psychotherapy must be a collaborative process between patient and therapist. You should take an active role in identifying and learning to resolve the emotional conflicts causing your stress. The principal therapeutic orientations that may be used—singly or, more likely, in combination—include the following:

- **Supportive therapy combined with insight-oriented treatment** works to reassure you that stress is temporary while helping you identify the psychiatric cause of your stress. The treatment helps you to achieve a more positive outlook and higher self-esteem. It also teaches intervention techniques, such as deep breathing, positive self-talk, and progressive muscle relaxation, that can be used to fight negative behaviors that lead to stress.
- **Cognitive/behavioral therapy** is based on the belief that all behavior (and perception) is learned and therefore can be unlearned. With your therapist, you look at how you perceive issues that trigger your stress, then structure and implement appropriate behavior modification by using various techniques. This therapy tries to bring about changes in your habits so that you correct the self-defeating thoughts that lead to stress.
- **Psychodynamic therapy** focuses on the subjective meaning of experience and uses therapy to explore, illuminate, and transform the way you experience yourself and others. This therapy examines the emotional issues that accompany stress and is generally used with those who deny the psychological reasons behind stress. This form will give you insight into psychiatric conflicts and feelings, help you clarify specific issues in your life, and help

you interpret your own problems as a prelude to your changing and taking responsibility for reducing your own stress.

If you don't know of a good psychiatrist, ask your primary care physician to suggest one or seek referrals from a local health or mental health agency or hospital. (Remember that hospital referrals are generally limited to those doctors on the hospital's staff.) Be certain you look for someone with a background in treating stress problems. To verify the board certification of any psychiatrist, call the American Board of Medical Specialties at 800-776-CERT.

SOCIAL, NONMEDICAL INTERVENTION

✓ *Try joining a stress management support group.*
Support groups can be economical, immediate ways to reduce stress. Experts say support groups reverse the isolation people feel in modern society, act as pseudofamilies where all players are equal, and naturally encourage members to air and share their vulnerable emotions. They offer a safe haven, a nonthreatening arena, where you can vent anger, voice fears, and start to let go of the negative emotions that cause stress by sharing experiences with those who have felt some of the same emotions. There's a possible added benefit, noted in the July 1995 *Consumer Reports on Health*: Researchers believe that stress reduction, such as that found in support groups for cancer patients, may actually help protect you against diseases such as cancer or help you live through it longer.

Look in local papers for listings of where and when self-help groups meet. Or contact the American Self-Help Clearinghouse, Northwest-Covenant Medical Center, 25 Pocono Road, Denville, NJ 07834 (201-625-7101), which maintains listings and publishes *The Self-Help Sourcebook.* If you're computer savvy, you may want to check out support groups on-line.

✔ Seek nonmedical psychological counseling for stress.

Nonmedical psychological counseling is done by a professional who is not an M.D. or a D.O. Psychologists have completed at least four years of graduate study in psychology at an accredited institution, generally hold a Ph.D. (doctor of philosophy) or Psy.D. (doctor of psychology) degree, and usually have a subspecialty in clinical or counseling psychology. In all states, they must be licensed to practice. While a psychologist may not prescribe drugs for a patient, a psychologist often works with a medical doctor when drugs are indicated.

Other nonphysician practitioners include clinical social workers, who have earned an M.S.W. (master of social work) degree following at least two years of directed postgraduate study. Qualified family therapists, those certified in marital and family therapy, should ideally have a master's degree in the kind of counseling they offer. Since only 25 states currently license family therapists, many less-than-qualified practitioners hang out a shingle with impunity. Therefore, it is worth your time to research and ask for credentials before you commit.

✔ *Participate in group counseling.*

If you can't tolerate one-on-one counseling, if you feel you'd do better mixing with others, or if you simply can't afford private counseling, group therapy may be for you. Group counseling models very closely on the self-help format, except that a trained mental health professional is involved, either as a group leader or as a facilitator. Groups of six to eight people generally meet weekly for 90 minutes, and when a member no longer needs the therapy, he or she leaves the group and is replaced by a newcomer.

Counseling groups can be single-focus, choosing to treat one issue or condition such as job-related stress, or mixed-focus, in which each participant may be there to solve a different type of interpersonal problem. Each format has particular strengths. In single-focus groups, a member can rely on others who know about the problem from personal experience, and those further along in counseling can inspire the newcomer with their progress. Mixed groups have strength in diversity. Members gain insights by playing off the group dynamic and the range of perspectives to overcome a number of problems.

Before you begin group therapy—or, frankly, any other type of therapy—first discuss with the counselor the specific goals you hope to reach. This will set a time frame against which both you and your counselor can evaluate your progress. In *The Consumer's Guide to Psychotherapy*, Jack Engler, Ph.D., and Daniel Coleman, Ph.D., state that many people suffering from stress find they benefit after as few as four sessions. Others need

six to eight sessions, and still others, who are the excep-
tions, may continue therapy for a much longer term.*

PHARMACOLOGICAL INTERVENTION

✓ *Avoid long-term use of OTC "remedies."*
Unlike other illnesses and conditions such as colds and
constipation, stress has no extensive drugstore shelf devoted to its treatment. That's because medications effective for treating anxiety are all psychoactive—affecting
normal mental functions—and are therefore restricted by
the Food and Drug Administration to a doctor's prescription. On the other hand, what are available are OTC
treatments for many stress *symptoms*: a full range of ant-
acids and bismuth mixtures for stomach distress; anal-
gesics and anti-inflammatory drugs for headaches,
arthritis, and other stress-prompted aches and pains; cold
formulas and medicated nasal sprays for stress-related
colds, sinus problems, and nasal allergy conditions; and
sleep aids for insomnia.

While few OTC medications make direct claims of
treating anxiety, in truth many of us use medications we
buy off the shelf for treating anxiety and stress symptoms. There's nothing wrong, of course, with taking an
occasional pain reliever for a tension headache or with
popping a few antacid tablets to offset the stressful effects that meeting had on your last meal. But they should
be taken only *occasionally*. OTC preparations, like their
prescriptive counterparts, are drugs, and they come with

---

*New York: Fireside, 1992.

a full menu of side effects, from dry mouth and drowsiness to impaired short-term memory and even, at times, visual hallucinations. Remember also that by treating stress symptoms—your body's distress signals—and disregarding stress itself, you are ignoring the real source of your problem and subjecting yourself to even greater damage.

✔ Know these classes of stress-related prescriptive drugs.

The prescriptive medications historically used to treat anxiety and stress are sedatives, anxiolytics (antianxiety drugs), and minor tranquilizers. In the past, most had severe negative side effects such as grogginess, and some were highly addictive. However, as they have evolved, antianxiety drugs have become more efficient, with fewer negative side effects.

Some current medications, namely the sedatives, are meant only as temporary treatments, not to be taken over a prolonged period. Other antianxiety drugs, including the monoamine oxidase inhibitors and selective serotonin reuptake inhibitors, are approved for long-term use. Here, in order of their arrival on the antianxiety scene, beginning with the older medications, are the major drug categories currently used to treat stress. (Examples of brand names are shown in parentheses.)

• **Benzodiazepines** (Librium, Valium, Xanax, Dalmane, Halcion) are usually helpful in short-term treatment related to defined circumstances, such as dealing with a recent emotional upheaval. They are intended to make a stressed person less anxious so that self-help can take effect and the person can get much-needed sleep.

They enhance the activity of some neurotransmitters—brain chemicals that reduce nerve-impulse transmissions and inhibit certain brain activity. Side effects are numerous, including addiction, drowsiness, and lack of coordination. They should be taken only for short periods (two weeks or less). Benzodiazepines are particularly worrisome for the elderly because these drugs are frequently overprescribed for lengthy periods. These medications are potentially lethal when mixed with alcohol.

• **Beta-blockers** (Inderal, Lopressor, Toprol-XL, Tenormin, Blocadren) lower high blood pressure, relieve angina, and stabilize irregular heartbeats. They are included under antianxiety medications because they block the brain's beta waves, which are associated with arousal and the stress hormone epinephrine. Beta-blockers are also used to control some migraine headaches, often a stress-related condition. Beta-blockers are not prescribed for those with breathing problems, because these drugs can cause airways to constrict. Other side effects include changes in heart rate, cold hands and feet, and depression. The biggest danger with beta-blockers is associated with abrupt withdrawal, which can precipitate heart attack, angina, and other serious side effects.

• **Monoamine oxidase inhibitors**, or MAOIs (Marplan, Nardil, Parnate), are antidepressants that increase the levels of the neurotransmitters epinephrine and serotonin (which is a calming chemical) by reducing the body's production of monoamine oxidase, an enzyme that normally breaks down these chemicals. Side effects include dizziness, dry mouth, and loss of sexual interest. MAOIs may also cause a serious reaction when mixed with alcoholic beverages or foods containing tyramine (for example, red wine and aged cheeses), resulting in a dangerous rise in blood pressure, nausea, possible confusion, psychotic symptoms, seizures, stroke, coma, and even death. MAOIs also interact with some OTC cold and allergy medicines, appetite suppressants, local anesthetics, insulin, medicines used to treat Parkinson's disease, and amphetamines. For this reason, MAOIs are often the last choice of treatment for reducing anxiety. They are typically prescribed for those who do not respond to tricyclic antidepressants, discussed next, and for cases of atypical depression.

• **Tricyclic antidepressants,** or **TCAs** (Tofranil, Elavil, Pamelor, Norpramin), were first prescribed in the 1950s and, until the development of selective serotonin reuptake inhibitors, were the top choice for treatment of major depressive disorders. They work by raising the levels of serotonin and norepinephrine in the brain by slowing the rate of absorption (or reuptake) of these two brain chemicals by nerve cells. Side effects vary but most commonly include dry mouth, constipation, and difficulty urinating, conditions known as anticholinergic side effects. Elderly users can also experience cognitive and memory difficulties. TCAs can prompt weight gain, dizziness, sweating, and fatigue, but such side effects often dissipate quickly or can be reduced by lowering the dosage or switching to another form of TCA. For those who report strong side effects or for whom TCAs appear not to work, MAOIs are sometimes substituted. TCAs are not addictive, but they can be lethal in overdose.

• **Selective serotonin reuptake inhibitors,** or **SSRIs** (Prozac, Zoloft, Paxil), are the newest major class of antidepressant. While TCAs inhibit the absorption of serotonin and norepinephrine, SSRIs treat depression and anxiety selectively by inhibiting the absorption (or reup-take) of serotonin only. Therefore, SSRIs lack the anti-cholinergic side effects of TCAs and the dietary restrictions of MAOIs, making them an attractive drug choice. Like other antidepressants, Prozac has been known to trigger manic episodes in those with personal or family histories of bipolar (manic-depressive) disor-der, but for various types of anxiety and other forms of depression, SSRIs have quickly become one of Amer-ica's most used drugs. Initial side effects of SSRIs may include nausea and diarrhea, anxiety, insomnia, head-ache, and rash, all likely to recede once the body has acclimated to the regimen. Overall, side effects known to date are the mildest of any antidepressant. Because the drugs are so new, little is known about possible long-term effects.

• **Other prescription drugs** used to treat depression and anxiety include venlafaxine (Effexor), trazodone (Desyrel), and bupropion (Wellbutrin). While they do not belong to any of the antidepressant classes, their ac-tivity partially resembles the SSRIs. Effexor, most like an SSRI, inhibits the absorption of norepinephrine as well as serotonin. Desyrel also works like an SSRI but has a different chemical composition. It is also the most sedating of the three drugs mentioned here, so it is gen-erally reserved for those with anxiety that exhibits agi-tation. Wellbutrin's effect on the brain is not yet fully understood, but it is believed to inhibit the absorption of serotonin, norepinephrine, and dopamine. Each of these drugs has the possibility of side effects, but for the most part, they are milder than most TCAs. They can be used long-term in the dosages prescribed with few side ef-fects.

USING PSYCHOACTIVE DRUGS

Psychoactive drugs have potentially miraculous properties, including the ability to restore debilitated stress sufferers to less anxious, more productive lives. However, these strong drugs alter brain chemistry, and some types may be addictive. They are often abused and may cause a range of negative side effects.

Never mix psychoactive drugs with alcohol, especially if you are taking any sedative or tranquilizer, since these medications depress the central nervous system. Combining this effect with that of alcohol, also a depressant, is enough to close down all of your bodily functions. If it's a temptation, lock up the liquor during your treatment or stash it with a friend. Alcohol never helps anyone under stress, and there have been many deaths and cerebral accidents resulting in coma among people who did not take this warning seriously—or who became so mellowed out on alcohol they forgot they had also taken a sedating drug.

The best advice is to treat all psychoactive drugs as the powerhouses they are. Use them in the way your doctor intended them to be used. Don't share them with anyone. And if you've been prescribed a drug that you've been told you should discontinue before your prescription runs out, follow those instructions—but be sure to follow doctor's orders if gradual withdrawal is indicated.

COMPLEMENTARY MEDICAL INTERVENTION

✔ *Explore alternative medicine.*

Alternative, or complementary, treatments—therapies not universally accepted by mainstream American medicine—hold great appeal. A survey reported in the January 28, 1993, issue of the *New England Journal of Medicine* indicated that one out of three adults questioned had used an "unconventional therapy" in the previous year, the same year that Americans spent some $13.7 billion on alternative techniques.

Complementary treatments such as acupuncture, yoga, massage, and nutrition—which enjoy widespread use in Europe, China, and Latin America—are accepted by numerous traditional physicians as effective stress therapy when used in combination with traditional treatments. Other alternative techniques, in their eyes, have yet to have their benefits clinically proved.

The following tips suggest some complementary approaches that have good records in the treatment of stress. As always, when dealing with a medical treatment of any kind, check first with your physician to be certain the combinations you are considering are complementary rather than counterproductive to any medical treatment you may be receiving.

ALTERNATIVE SYSTEMS OF MEDICAL PRACTICE

• **Acupuncture,** an ancient Chinese medical system, follows the principle that disease results from an imbalance in the body's energy, called "chi." In acupuncture, thin needles are inserted just below the skin along paths known as meridians, the "energy highways" through which acupuncturists believe energy and blood flow throughout the body. Through acupuncture, the balance between the life forces of yin and yang is restored, therefore restoring health. Studies indicate that acupuncture releases endorphins that counteract pain and diminish the effect of the stress hormones. Acupuncture has had good immediate results with stress reduction, though relief is not always long-lasting without additional treatments. Acupuncturists are not licensed in every state. Check your state health department to learn your state's licensing laws.

• **Acupressure** is the older cousin of acupuncture. Modern acupressure evolved from an ancient Chinese healing art in which fingers press key points on the surface of the skin to stimulate the body's natural healing abilities. Acupressure proponents say that when the points are pressed, muscular tension is released, circulation improves, and the body's life force to aid healing is promoted. Acupressure is also thought to inhibit pain signals to the brain. Michael Reed Gach, one of America's leading acupressure authorities, identifies in *Acupressure's Potent Points* eight "potent pressure points" for relieving stress-related frustration and irritation.*

• **Ayurveda,** or **Ayurvedic medicine,** is the traditional, holistic medicine of India and the oldest of the healing arts. It employs meditation, herbals, and nutrition to achieve a balance of the body's energy and a "harmonious collective consciousness." Ayurveda is often

---

*New York: Bantam, 1990.

used in the treatment of chronic conditions affected by stress, including arthritis, eczema, high blood pressure, sinusitis, and headaches. Ayurveda has been popularized in the United States by best-selling author Deepak Chopra, M.D. Although Ayurvedic healers are not licensed in any state, some 200 M.D.'s and D.O.'s are trained in Ayurveda and incorporate Ayurvedic principles into their practices.

• **Naturopathy** is an American form of medicine, first popular in the 19th century, that draws from several medical systems, including acupuncture, nutrition, pharmacology, manipulative therapies, and botanical medicine. Naturopathic doctors champion medicines with all-natural ingredients and practice preventive medicine by working to enhance the body's healing abilities. Naturopathy is considered more effective in the treatment of chronic conditions such as stress than in the treatment of infections or illnesses, which may respond better to a biomedical approach. Only a few states license naturopathic physicians, but the American Association of Naturopathic Physicians (AANP) does certify practitioners. The 1,000-plus certified naturopathic doctors practicing in the United States hold an N.D. (doctor of naturopathic medicine) degree, which is granted upon successful completion of a four-year program at one of the country's several accredited naturopathic colleges. To determine whether a naturopathic doctor is certified, write the AANP at 2366 Eastlake Avenue, Suite 322, Seattle, WA 98102, or call 206-323-7610.

MEDITATIVE MOVEMENT THERAPIES
Meditative movement therapies invoke the high consciousness of meditation along with measured, calming

body movements. Research has shown that these movement therapies can claim excellent results in helping to relieve stress.

• **Yoga,** which means "union of disciplines," combines a series of complex stretching exercises with deep breathing, meditation, and postures (*asanas*). Yoga is thought to restore harmony and balance between the body and the soul, and studies show that yoga can lower blood pressure, in all probability by slowing the production of epinephrine while the mind is in the meditative state. There is no license required for yoga instructors, but it is important to find a practitioner who is competent and has some training in anatomy and physiology. Some organizations do offer certification. To find a certified teacher, write the Himalayan International Institute of Yoga at R.R. 1, P.O. Box 400, Honesdale, PA 18431, or call 800-822-4547 or 717-253-5551.

• **Tai chi** centers on the same fundamental principle as Chinese healing therapies: achieving harmony so that energy may flow freely. This meditative exercise uses a full range of motion and consists of slow, well-ordered, "flowing" body movements designed to promote physical strength, mental clarity, and emotional serenity. A license is not required to teach exercise and movement therapies, but tai chi and qigong (an exercise therapy similar to tai chi) are best learned from knowledgeable, trained instructors. Contact local Ys, health clubs, or spas to find out where these therapies are offered in your area.

MANUAL HEALING METHODS

• **Massage therapy** can effectively reduce stress. More than 100 different kinds of massage therapies exist, and all consist of manipulating the body's soft tissues to treat various diseases and conditions. Acupressure and aromatherapy are forms of massage, as are Swedish massage, trigger-point (shiatsu) therapy, and reflexology (which uses pressure points on the feet). Massage increases circulation, reduces tightness in involuntary muscles (blood vessels, heart, gastrointestinal tract) and voluntary muscles, stimulates the release of pain-relieving endorphins, and lowers stress hormone levels. Licensing of massage therapists is spotty: Some states require licenses, others don't. Additional training is recommended for some special forms of massage. Spas, local health clubs, and salons usually keep a list of massage therapists in the area. You may want to call the National Certification Board for Therapeutic Massage and Bodywork at 800-296-0664 for names of bodywork therapists they've certified. You can also call the American Massage Therapy Association at 312-761-AMTA for more information.

• **Chiropractic therapy** is a distinctly American form of medical therapy that involves treating the whole person, rather than the disease, with a healing touch and manipulation of the body's bones, muscles, and soft tissues. According to chiropractic theory, the body is controlled by the nervous system, and various joint dislocations (subluxations) throw the body out of balance, resulting in disease. The drug-free therapy focuses on realignment of the spine through manipulation; once balance of the spine and nervous system is restored, the body is able to heal itself, says this theory. Many patients who have sought stress and tension relief, treatment of lower back and other muscle pain, and relief from a variety of painful chronic conditions through chiropractic therapy have been satisfied with the results. This therapy, which is preventive as well as healing, also employs hydrotherapy, electrical stimulation, ultrasound, massage, nutrition, and exercise. Chiropractors are not medical doctors and can't write prescriptions or perform surgery, but mandatory licensing in all states requires that they hold a doctor of chiropractic (D.C.) degree.

• **Osteopathic therapy** is an American form of therapy that uses two techniques-manipulation of the musculoskeletal system and palpation, or touching the body-to locate external signs of internal problems. Osteopathic theory holds that the body's mechanical structure and function are interdependent and that disease occurs when these are out of sync. Though they both use manipulation, osteopathy has been more readily accepted than chiropractic therapy in the American medical mainstream because osteopaths receive medical education similar to that of an M.D. and may write prescriptions and perform surgery. A doctor of osteopathy (D.O.) degree requires education at a four-year college accredited by the American Association of Colleges of Osteopathic Medicine. D.O.'s are required to be licensed in all states.

MIND-BODY INTERVENTION

• **Hypnosis** by a certified hypnotherapist (not to be confused with self-hypnosis, a relaxation strategy) is another approach to stress relief that some find successful. For years hypnosis has been incorrectly associated with dramatic trances and the surrender of total control to a therapist, but neither stereotype is accurate.

Hypnosis involves first discussing the stress source (for example, fear of speaking in front of a group) and hypnosis goals (to be able to detach public speaking from the fear) with the therapist. The therapist then hypnotizes the person by initiating a relaxation response and helping the person shift thoughts away from everyday activities and toward inner thoughts and sensations. While the person is in this relaxed state and the mind is most open to suggestion, the therapist asks the patient to imagine he or she is experiencing a situation that causes stress and is responding in a relaxed manner. After perhaps four or five more sessions, the rehearsed mental image is said to transfer to real-life behavior. The dividend of such instruction is that the person soon learns to shift into the deep relaxation state at will, a handy skill that helps reduce stress. Many people call themselves hypnotherapists, but not all are qualified. Verify the certification of a qualified professional by contacting the American Society of Clinical Hypnosis. Send a self-addressed, stamped envelope to 2200 East Devon Avenue, Suite 291, Des Plaines, IL 60018, or call 847-297-3317.

BIOELECTROMAGNETIC THERAPY

• **TENS,** which stands for transcutaneous electrical nerve stimulation, is a high-tech complementary therapy in which low-voltage alternating current (AC) is passed through a painful area of the body via electrodes. The mild current stimulates production of painkilling endorphins while blocking the transmission of pain and stress impulses. Used extensively by chiropractors, TENS helps relieve tension (and migraine) headaches and back, neck, joint, and other muscle pains. A treatment generally lasts from 10 to 30 minutes. Relief is usually immediate but temporary. Clinical experimentation with TENS apparatuses using stronger direct current (DC) has shown some success in achieving more lasting relief, measured in months rather than hours.

These tips for the prevention and treatment of stress have provided you with helpful insights and techniques for controlling your own anxiety. Remember that just as it took a long time for you to build up to a level of stress that you consider unhealthy, learning and implementing effective stress management techniques in your life is not an overnight process. But if you're serious about stress management, we promise you it will change your life for the better.

APPENDIX

STRESS SELF-TESTS

GIVE YOURSELF A STRESS TEST

The following test, developed by researchers at Carnegie Mellon University, provides a rough measure of how much stress you're experiencing. For each question, circle the appropriate number.

In the past month, how often have you felt:	Never	Almost never	Some-times	Fairly often	Very often
Upset because of something that happened unexpectedly?	0	1	2	3	4
Unable to control the important things in your life?	0	1	2	3	4
Unable to cope with all the things you had to do?	0	1	2	3	4

In the past month, how often have you felt:	Never	Almost never	Some-times	Fairly often	Very often
Angered because of things that were beyond your control?	0	1	2	3	4
That difficulties were piling up so high you could not overcome them?	0	1	2	3	4
Confident about your abilities to handle your personal problems?	4	3	2	1	0
That things were going your way?	4	3	2	1	0
Able to control irritations in your life?	4	3	2	1	0
That you were on top of things?	4	3	2	1	0

Total score: _____

The higher your total score on the test, the greater your stress level. The average score for the general population is 14 for women, 12 for men.

Source: Cohen, Sheldon, Tom Kamarck, and Robin Mermelstein, "A Global Measure of Perceived Stress," *Journal of Health and Social Behavior*, vol. 24, 385–396, 1983. Reprinted by permission of the American Sociological Association.

IS STRESS CURRENTLY AFFECTING YOU PHYSICALLY?

Mark "yes" for those symptoms you experience more than once weekly. If monthly, answer "sometimes," and if less frequently than monthly, answer "no."

	Yes	Some-times	No
Is your sleep disturbed by any of the following?	___	___	___
a. difficulty getting to sleep	___	___	___
b. waking frequently in the night	___	___	___
c. waking in the early hours, unable to sleep again	___	___	___
Are you experiencing sexual difficulties (such as impotence or lack of desire for sex)?	___	___	___
Do you have difficulty sitting still without fidgeting?	___	___	___
Do you have headaches?	___	___	___
Do you bite your nails?	___	___	___
Do you feel unusually tired?	___	___	___
Do you have frequent indigestion, such as heartburn?	___	___	___
Do you crave food other than at mealtimes?	___	___	___
Do you have no appetite at mealtimes?	___	___	___
Is bowel function erratic-sometimes constipated, sometimes very loose?	___	___	___
Do you sweat for no obvious reason?	___	___	___
Do you have any "tics," such as touching the face, hair, or moustache repeatedly?	___	___	___

	Yes	Some-times	No
Do you frequently feel nauseated?	___	___	___
Do you ever faint or have dizzy spells without obvious cause?	___	___	___
Do you feel breathless and tight-chested when not exerting yourself?	___	___	___
Do you cry or feel the desire to cry?	___	___	___
Are you suffering from high blood pressure?	___	___	___
Do you feel obligated to take a drink to "unwind"?	___	___	___
Do you smoke to calm your nerves?	___	___	___

If you answered "yes" to two or more of these questions (two "sometimes" answers are equal to one "yes"), then you are almost certainly feeling the effects of stress, and it is time to take appropriate action. Some of the above symptoms can arise from other causes, but usually these are combined with stress factors. In the absence of organic disease, all such symptoms are remediable by stress management.

Source: Chaitow, Leon. *Stress.* London: Thorsons, 1995. Reprinted by permission of the publisher.

LIFE CHANGE INDEX

To rate how much stress you are experiencing in your life, add up the numbers listed for life events you have undergone within the past year. If you score more than 200, you have a 50 percent chance of becoming seriously ill from stress; a score of 300 or more raises your chance of illness to 80 percent.

Life event	Score
1. Death of a spouse	100
2. Divorce	73
3. Marital separation	65
4. Jail term	63
5. Death of a close family member	63
6. Personal injury or illness	53
7. Marriage	50
8. Being fired	47
9. Marital reconciliation	45
10. Retirement	45
11. Change in the health of a family member	44
12. Pregnancy	40
13. Sexual difficulties	39
14. Having a baby	39
15. Business readjustment	39
16. Change in financial state	38
17. Death of a close friend	37
18. Change to a different line of work	36
19. Change in the number of arguments with spouse	35
20. Mortgage large in relation to income	31
21. Foreclosure of mortgage or loan	30
22. Change in responsibilities at work	29
23. Son or daughter leaving home	29
24. Trouble with in-laws	29
25. Outstanding personal achievement	28
26. Spouse beginning or ending work	26
27. Beginning or ending school	26
28. Change in living conditions	25
29. Change in personal habits	24
30. Trouble with boss	23
31. Change in work hours or conditions	20
32. Change in residence	20

Life event	Score
33. Change in schools.	20
34. Change in church activities	19
35. Change in recreation	19
36. Change in social activities.	18
37. Small mortgage in relation to income	17
38. Change in sleeping habits	16
39. Change in number of family get-togethers	15
40. Change in eating habits	13
41. Vacation.	13
42. Christmas.	12
43. Minor violation of the law	11

Source: Holmes and Rahe, "Social Readjustment Rating Scale," *Psychosomatic Research*, vol. 11. Oxford, England: Pergamon, 1967. Reprinted by permission of the publisher.

GLOSSARY

Antioxidant: A molecule that helps limit potentially harmful oxidative reactions by neutralizing free radicals. Free radicals are molecular fragments that attempt to steal electrons from other molecules. An antioxidant donates an electron to the free radical, thereby neutralizing it. Nutrients that act as antioxidants include vitamins A, C, and E, beta-carotene, and selenium.

Benzodiazepines: A group of drugs that reduces anxiety by enhancing the activity of neurotransmitters, the brain chemicals that reduce nerve-impulse transmissions and inhibit certain brain activity.

Beta-blocker: A drug used primarily to lower high blood pressure, relieve angina, and stabilize irregular heartbeats. It is considered an antianxiety medication because it blocks the brain's beta waves, associated with arousal, and the stress hormone epinephrine.

Breakdown: A condition that results when a person's ability to cope with the ordinary demands of life is damaged by stress. Symptoms include fatigue, irritability, and fear. It can result in permanent vulnerability to stress.

Burnout: A stress-related condition that results from prolonged stress. Symptoms include lethargy, alienation, indifference to activities, and lack of satisfaction.

Clinical social worker: A mental health professional, typically with a master's degree in social work, who is trained to offer psychotherapy.

Cognitive/behavioral therapy: A psychotherapeutic approach based on the belief that all behavior (and perception) is learned and can therefore be unlearned. This therapy tries to bring about changes in behavior and attitude and teaches coping techniques.

Complementary medicine: An alternative therapy, such as osteopathy, chiropractic therapy, or acupuncture, used in addition to traditional medical care.

Cortisol: A hormone that is secreted during stress of any kind.

Depression: Persistent feelings of sadness, despair, and discouragement, which may be a symptom of an underlying mental or physical disorder.

Endorphins: Compounds that affect parts of the brain that process information about pain, emotion, and feelings. They are sometimes called the feel-good hormones.

Epinephrine: A hormone that is secreted during stress of any kind. It is also known as adrenaline.

Fight-or-flight: Another term for the stress response. It indicates that the response is prepared by the body in order to face the stressor head-on (fight) or to escape the stressor (flight).

Monoamine oxidase inhibitors (MAOIs): A group of drugs that increases the levels of the neurotransmitters epinephrine and serotonin by reducing production of the enzyme monoamine oxidase, which normally breaks down these chemicals.

Norepinephrine: A stress hormone triggered by a protein containing the amino acid tyrosine. It is also known as noradrenaline.

Psychiatrist: A physician who specializes in the diagnosis and treatment of mental or psychiatric disorders.

Psychoactive drug: A drug that affects the mind or behavior.

Psychodynamic therapy: A psychotherapeutic approach that focuses on the underlying drives and desires that determine behavior.

Psychologist: A person with a doctoral degree in psychology (Ph.D. or Psy.D.) and training in counseling, psychotherapy, and psychological testing.

Psychotherapeutic counseling: Therapy employing psychological methods ranging from psychoanalysis to behavioral modification.

Selective serotonin reuptake inhibitors (SSRIs): Antidepressant agents that treat depression and anxiety by inhibiting the reuptake (or absorption) of serotonin.

Serotonin: A neurotransmitter found in the brain that has been linked to calm feelings.

Stress: An event or situation that disrupts a person's healthy mental and physical well-being and results in emotional or physical tension, or the state of emotional or physical tension that results from such a disruption.

Stress hormones: Chemicals, including cortisol and epinephrine, produced by the brain in times of stress to trigger the preparation of the body's systems.

Stressor: An internal or external cause of stress.

Stress response: The physiological process that automatically occurs in the body in response to stress: recognition of stress; preparation by the body's systems to meet stress; successful resistance or adaptation to stress; and exhaustion (if exposure to stress is prolonged).

Supportive therapy: Short-term therapy that emphasizes supporting, rather than changing, the person who is depressed or anxious.

Tricyclic antidepressants (TCAs): A type of antidepressant that raises the levels of serotonin and norepinephrine in the brain by slowing their rate of absorption (or reuptake) by nerve cells.

INDEX